Clinical Cases
in Obstetrics,
y
and women's
Health

7
Day
Loan

NOTICE

Medicine is an ever-changing science. As new research and clinical experience broaden our knowledge, changes in treatment and drug therapy are required. The editors and the publisher of this work have checked with sources believed to be reliable in their efforts to provide information that is complete and generally in accord with the standards accepted at the time of publication. However, in view of the possibility of human error or changes in medical sciences, neither the editors, nor the publisher, nor any other party who has been involved in the preparation or publication of this work warrants that the information contained herein is in every respect accurate or complete. Readers are encouraged to confirm the information contained herein with other sources. For example, and in particular, readers are advised to check the product information sheet included in the package of each drug they plan to administer to be certain that the information contained in this book is accurate and that changes have not been made in the recommended dose or in the contraindications for administration. This recommendation is of particular importance in connection with new or infrequently used drugs.

CLINICAL CASES SERIES

Clinical Cases in Obstetrics, Gynaecology and Women's Health

CAROLINE DE COSTA

PAUL HOWAT

Department of Obstetrics and Gynaecology
James Cook University School of Medicine,
Cairns Campus

The **McGraw·Hill** Companies

Sydney New York San Francisco Auckland
Bangkok Bogotá Caracas Hong Kong
Kuala Lumpur Lisbon London Madrid
Mexico City Milan New Delhi San Juan
Seoul Singapore Taipei Toronto

Mc Graw Hill **Medical**

First published 2007

Text © 2007 Caroline de Costa and Paul Howat
Illustrations and design © 2007 McGraw-Hill Australia Pty Ltd
Additional owners of copyright are acknowledged on the Acknowledgments page.

National Library of Australia Cataloguing-in-Publication data:

De Costa, Caroline, 1947– .
   Clinical cases in obstetrics, gynaecology and women's health.
   Includes index.
   ISBN 9780074716403.
   ISBN 0 074 71640 9.

   1. Obstetrics—Case studies. 2. Gynecology—Case studies. 3. Women—Health and hygiene. I. Howat, Paul. II. Title. (Series: Clinical cases in emergency medicine).
   618

Published in Australia by
McGraw-Hill Australia Pty Ltd
Level 2, 82 Waterloo Road, North Ryde NSW 2113
Publishing Manager: Jo Munnelly
Acquisitions Editor: Nicole Meehan
Production Editor: Samantha Miles
Editor: Carolyn Pike
Permissions Editor: Jared Dunn
Proofreader: Tim Learner
Indexer: Glenda Browne
Designer (cover and interior): Jan Schmoeger, Designpoint
Illustrators: Nives Porcellato and Andrew Craig
Printed by 1010 Printing International Limited, China

Contents

Contents by subject matter

Acknowledgments

We wish to thank all the staff of the Women's Health Unit and the Operating Suite of Cairns Base Hospital, with whom we have worked over the past 15 years, and who have taught us much of what we have included in this book. In particular we thank Paul McNamara for his assistance with the case study concerned with post-natal depression. We are also grateful to Josie Valese of James Cook University School of Medicine for her invaluable advice about IT matters.

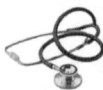

About the authors

Caroline de Costa is Professor of Obstetrics and Gynaecology at James Cook University School of Medicine, Cairns Campus.

Paul Howat is Director of Obstetrics and Gynaecology at Cairns Base Hospital, Cairns, and Adjunct Senior Lecturer at James Cook University School of Medicine.

Introduction

This book is addressed to the medical student following the core curriculum in Australia and New Zealand, the junior doctor at resident or house officer level, and the doctor caring for women in general practice, family planning practice or in a women's health clinic.

Although the book broadly covers the whole syllabus for the medical student, and the whole range of obstetric and gynaecological problems likely to come into the path of the busy junior hospital doctor or general practitioner, it is not a textbook providing simply a list of differential diagnoses and treatments. Our approach has developed from our experience teaching problem-based learning scenarios (PBLs) to clinical students from James Cook University School of Medicine. PBLs introduce students to typical clinical situations and then encourage those students to think about how they would take appropriate histories, examine, investigate and finally treat their patients. In this book, by using case histories that are more developed and complex than most of our PBLs, we aim to show readers in greater detail how women may present with particular conditions, and demonstrate what should take place in the way of consultation, investigations and treatment. However, by questioning our readers as we go along we also hope to encourage them to think about why they would choose a certain clinical course of action and to base their decisions firmly on current scientific evidence. In addition to the purely clinical aspects of the cases, emotional, social and psychological aspects of the care of each woman is described. We expect that the book will be used in conjunction with existing standard texts.

Each of the 41 case histories commences with a straightforward description following a woman through the clinical presentation of a particular condition. Along the way, important points in clinical examination and diagnosis, complications, investigations and management are incorporated into the text as a conversation with the reader, and essential points are highlighted in boxes. Finally, one or more 'clinical pearls' are appended—we hope that these gems will lodge permanently in the brain of the reader as they are facts that should never be forgotten when dealing with the particular condition. References for the information provided can be found at the end of each case history together with suggestions for further reading.

At the end of the book are 30 multiple choice questions for self-testing.

In the chapters dealing with obstetrics and gynaecology we address the reader as a house officer or resident charged with the daily (and nightly) care of patients in a busy urban hospital setting. Being ourselves practitioners in a rural area, we have at times included tips for those junior doctors faced with obstetric or gynaecological problems in a smaller metropolitan or rural setting—facilities for care and the advice of senior practitioners may be more limited in such surroundings and different care paths may be more appropriate.

In the section dealing with women's health, we address the reader as a general practitioner in an urban or rural setting, in a women's health clinic or in a family planning clinic. We hope the transfer from one clinical situation to another will prove understandable to the general reader. We have found this method of direct conversation, about situations they will shortly face as junior doctors, very acceptable to the medical students of JCU School of Medicine whom we teach daily at the campus in Cairns.

Common abbreviations

ACE	angiotensin-converting enzyme
AFI	amniotic fluid index
ARM	artificial rupture of the membranes
BMI	body mass index
BP	blood pressure
BPD	biparietal diameter
BSL	blood sugar level
BSO	bilateral salpingo-oophorectomy
CA-125	cancer antigen 125
CASA	cancer-associated serum antigen
CIN	cervical intraepithelial neoplasia
COCP	combined oral contraceptive pill
CRL	crown–rump length
CT	computed tomography
CTG	cardiotocography
CVP	central venous pressure
CVS	chorionic villus sampling
D&C	dilatation and curettage
DHEAS	dehydroepiandrosterone sulfate
DMPA	depot medroxyprogesterone acetate
DVT	deep venous thrombosis
ECV	external cephalic version
EDC	expected date of confinement
EDD	expected date of delivery
EFW	estimated fetal weight
ESR	erythrocyte sedimentation rate
EUA	examination under anaesthesia
FBC	full blood count
fFn	fetal fibronectin
FL	femur length
FNT	fetal nuchal translucency

FSH	follicle stimulating hormone
FTA-AbS	fluorescent treponemal antibodies
GBS	group B *Streptococcus*
GDM	gestational diabetes mellitus
GTT	glucose tolerance test
Hb	haemoglobin
HbA$_{1c}$	glycosylated haemoglobin
HCV	hepatitis C virus
HIV	human immunodeficiency virus
HPV	human papillomavirus
HSG	hysterosalpingogram
HSIL	high-grade squamous intraepithelial lesion
HSV	herpes simplex virus
IM	intramuscular
IUCD	intrauterine contraceptive device
IUGR	intrauterine growth restriction
IV	intravenous
IVF	in-vitro fertilisation
LBC	liquid-based cytology
LDH	lactate dehydrogenase
LFT	liver function test
LH	luteinising hormone
LLETZ	large loop excision of the transformation zone
LMP	last menstrual period
LMWH	low-molecular-weight heparin
LSIL	low-grade squamous intraepithelial lesion
MRI	magnetic resonance imaging
MSU	midstream urine
NHMRC	National Health and Medical Research Council
NSAIDs	non-steroidal anti-inflammatory drugs
PAPP-A	pregnancy-associated plasma protein
PCOS	polycystic ovarian syndrome
PGF$_{2\alpha}$	prostaglandin F$_{2\alpha}$
PID	pelvic inflammatory disease
RPR	rapid plasma reagin
SSRI	selective serotonin reuptake inhibitor
STI	sexually transmitted infection
TAH	total abdominal hysterectomy
TFT	thyroid function test
TPHA	*Treponema pallidum* haemagglutination antibody
TPL	'threatened' preterm labour

TVUSS	transvaginal ultrasound scans
UFH	unfractionated heparin
USS	ultrasound scan
UTI	urinary tract infection
VBAC	vaginal birth after caesarean section
VDRL	Venereal Disease Research Laboratories
VIN	vulval intraepithelial neoplasia
VTE	venous thromboembolism
β-HCG	beta-human chorionic gonadotrophin

Part 1
Guidelines

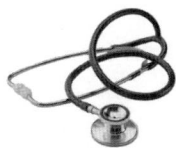

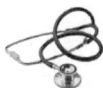

Taking an obstetric or gynaecological history

The principles underlying history taking from women presenting with symptoms and signs suggesting obstetric or gynaecological conditions do not differ from those applied to history taking in every other field of medicine. However, we do emphasise two points.

1 Around every womb there is a woman—although the presenting complaint may direct you immediately to the genital tract (e.g. major vaginal bleeding), do not neglect other body systems or the psychological and emotional aspects of the woman's presentation.
2 Remember that all women of reproductive age should be regarded as possibly pregnant until proved otherwise—be cautious about ruling out pregnancy on history alone.

Taking a gynaecological history

- Presenting complaint—what has brought the woman along to see you (e.g. pain, bleeding, failure to conceive, urinary incontinence, sexual difficulties)?
- History of presenting complaint—how long have the symptoms bothered the woman?; how severe are they?; any related symptoms? This history may include questions about menstrual disturbance, bleeding problems, premenstrual symptoms, lower abdominal pain or dyspareunia, infertility, pelvic floor dysfunction, menopausal symptoms, and so on.
- General gynaecological history—note the age of the woman, LMP, date of last Pap smear, any breast screening, contraception, parity, previous gynaecological surgery, previous gynaecological investigations and results. A reminder of the need for regular well woman checks, Pap smears and mammograms (in women over 40 years of age) is almost always useful.

- General medical and surgical history—history of any sexually transmitted infections, obstetric history, family history, any current medications, allergies.
- Social history—family support, cigarette smoking, use of alcohol and recreational drugs, work situation.

We recommend that when concluding your history and before commencing your examination of the woman you ask a broad question such as 'Are there any other things about you or your health that you think I should know?'. This may enable the woman to speak about personal matters that are worrying her. It also provides you with the assurance that from a medicolegal point of view you have endeavoured to obtain all relevant information.

Make sure that you document the history legibly and with sufficient detail.

Taking an obstetric history

In many cases, as a general practitioner or junior doctor consulted for the first time by a pregnant woman presenting with an apparent complication of pregnancy, you will have accessible copies of hospital booking notes or a shared care card containing much relevant information. However, with or without this pre-existing information we recommend you note the following points:

- presenting complaint (e.g. pain, bleeding, rupture of membranes, absence of fetal movements)—the duration and severity of the symptoms should be recorded
- age of woman, her gravidity and parity; date on which her last menstrual period (LMP) began; her expected date of confinement (EDC) by dates; results of any ultrasound scans (USS) that may have been performed; previous contraception; last Pap smear
- past obstetric history, including all full-term pregnancies, vaginal births, caesarean sections, miscarriages, abortions, ectopic pregnancies, perinatal deaths, preterm labours, postnatal complications
- past gynaecological, surgical and medical history, including any sexually transmitted infections, any current medications, allergies
- cigarette smoking, alcohol and recreational drug use, social history (i.e. family support, work situation), family history

Again, make sure that all documentation is complete and legible.

Conducting an examination

Examination of the adult gynaecological patient

1   Relevant general examination—assessment of vital signs appropriate to the case (pulse, BP, temperature) and examination of other systems and organs (heart, lungs, breasts in particular) should be conducted as indicated.

2   Examination of the abdomen—inspection for scars of previous surgery, striae, obvious masses; palpation for tenderness, masses, whether arising from the pelvis or elsewhere, ascites. Do not omit to palpate for an enlarged liver or spleen.

3   Vaginal examination—note that this is not always necessary at the initial visit. If a vaginal examination is performed, you need to be clear in your mind why you are doing the examination and what you are looking for. The vast majority of women find vaginal examination invasive to some degree, uncomfortable at best. However, this should not serve as an excuse for not performing a vaginal examination if it is required. This excuse is too often used by junior doctors and general practitioners who perhaps feel uncomfortable or uncertain in this situation. Serious pathology, in particular cervical cancer, can be missed because this examination has been avoided due to specious reasoning. It is essential that the woman herself understands why you are performing the examination, what you are looking for, has consented verbally to the procedure and is given the result insofar as is possible when the examination is concluded. It is our practice and recommendation to have a female chaperone present for all breast and genital examinations, irrespective of the gender of the practitioner, however we appreciate that this is not possible in all practices. The woman should be able to undress and dress again in privacy and should only have the results of your findings and other matters explained and discussed when she is fully dressed and sitting back in the consulting room. It is inappropriate for a fully dressed doctor

(or other health professional) to be holding a discussion with a partly dressed woman lying on a gynaecological couch.

Vaginal examination is usually conducted with the woman in the dorsal position. Examination of the vulva (looking for erythema, atrophic changes, swellings, suspicious lesions) should be performed prior to the vaginal examination itself.

4 Speculum examination—it is generally recommended that this be performed before a bimanual vaginal examination if a Pap smear is to be taken to avoid displacing cells from the surface of the cervix. However, a gentle one-finger vaginal examination prior to passing the speculum is permissible—this enables you to know whether the cervix is lying posteriorly high in the vagina because the uterus is anteverted (the case in about 75% of women), or is more anterior because the uterus is retroverted (as it is in the remaining 25%). Where the cervix lies anteriorly, the speculum should be gently passed more in this direction. The procedure for conducting a speculum examination is as follows:

   • Warm the speculum. A gel-type lubricant may be used if a Pap smear is not being taken, however, warm water is usually a sufficient lubricant.
   • Sometimes, placing the patient's fists or a cushion underneath her buttocks will assist in making the examination more comfortable and the cervix more easily visible.
   • Note the appearance of the cervix—normal/abnormal?
   • Note the presence and characteristics of any vaginal discharge.
   • The left lateral position using Sims' speculum may give a more complete view when assessing prolapse.

5 Bimanual examination—this is normally performed with two fingers of the dominant hand intra-vaginally and the other hand palpating the lower abdomen, so that the fundus of an anteverted uterus can be balloted between the two hands, and any pelvic masses examined likewise. (Examination couches are frequently placed against the left-hand wall of the room so left-handed practitioners may need to conduct vaginal examinations with the right hand.) Using the two hands, the following features should be assessed:

   • uterus—size, position, shape, consistency, any tenderness, mobility
   • adnexae—presence or absence of any masses or tenderness (note normal ovaries are not usually palpable as discrete masses but may be tender if pressed between the examining hands)

- utero–sacral nodularity/tenderness/tethering, which may suggest endometriosis.

Examination of the pregnant woman

As with gynaecological patients, a general physical examination should not be neglected. The woman should be made as comfortable as possible; in late pregnancy it may be appropriate either to ask the woman to turn slightly towards you or to place a pillow or wedge beneath her so that the weight of the fetus does not obstruct venous return, leading to syncope. You must also explain to the woman what you are doing and why.

Blood pressure should always be taken, preferably in a standard manner. In our clinic we take blood pressure in the right arm with the patient sitting up on the couch, her feet resting on a stool. If the circumference of the upper arm is greater than 27 cm, a large cuff should be used.

Abdominal examination

1 Inspection

- Is the abdomen distended?
- Are there any scars? Are there needle marks from the use of subcutaneous injections, such as for insulin or anticoagulants? Striae from the current or previous pregnancies may be apparent.

2 Palpation

The uterus is palpable in the abdomen from 12 weeks of pregnancy. Its size, shape, consistency and any tenderness should be noted. Fetal parts are palpable from 24–28 weeks dependent on the thickness of the abdominal wall. From 28 weeks onwards the lie of the fetus (relationship of the longitudinal axis of the fetus to the longitudinal axis of the uterus) can be determined. The nature of the presenting part (that part of the fetus lying in the lower uterine segment) may also be evident on palpation from 28 weeks onwards although again this depends on the degree of thickness of the abdominal wall—it may be difficult on occasion to confidently distinguish breech presentation from cephalic even for experienced practitioners. With cephalic presentations the degree of descent of the fetal head in relation to the pelvic brim should be noted from 36 weeks gestation onwards.

Note should also be made of any abdominal tenderness or enlargement of other abdominal organs.

3 Measurement

- Measure the pregnant uterus in centimetres from the symphysis pubis to the top of the uterus—this gives the fundal height. This examination is done from 20 weeks' gestation, when the fundus will be approximately level with the umbilicus. The height (in cm) should correspond approximately with the gestation in weeks.

4 Auscultation

- This is mainly of use in obstetrics for identifying the fetal heart sounds, which is most easily heard with an electronic Doppler device; a standard stethoscope is unable to detect fetal heart sounds easily.

Part 2
Clinical Cases in General Practice

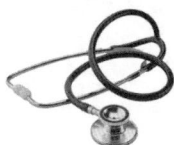

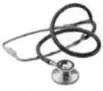

Case 1
Kate presents for a well-woman check …

Kate is a 19-year-old university student who has made an appointment to see you in general practice for a well-woman check and to discuss contraception. You have been Kate's family doctor since she was 10 years old. Apart from normal childhood illnesses Kate has always been in good health.

At the age of 14 she presented with primary dysmenorrhoea for which you prescribed mefenamic acid, after normal findings at a general physical examination. This was effective for 2 years but at the age of 16 Kate developed more severe dysmenorrhoea. Examination at that time was again unremarkable and Kate had never been sexually active. She was commenced on a combined oral contraceptive pill (COCP)—ethinyloestradiol 30 µg, levonorgestrel 150 µg—and this has completely controlled her period-related pain ever since. When Kate presented for her annual prescription about 1 year ago she stated that she had been sexually active for the past year. You reminded her about safe sex and she replied that she and her boyfriend were using condoms. She asked you about regular Pap smears and you advised her that she should return for the first of these in 12 months. You explained to her the national guidelines for Pap smear screening.

All women over the age of 18 who have ever had sex and who have a cervix should have regular Pap smears every 2 years, even if they no longer have sex. They should start between the ages of 18 and 20 years, or 1 or 2 years after first having sex, whichever is later, and continue up to the age of 70. At age 70, if previous Pap smears have been normal their doctor may advise them that they no longer need Pap smears. Cervical cancer is one of the most preventable of all cancers. It is the eighth most common cancer in Australian women. Up to 90% of squamous cell carcinoma can be prevented if cell changes can be detected and treated early.

How do you commence your consultation with Kate?

Kate reports that she is well. She has continued on the COCP and has no concerns with this but she does wonder whether it is safe to continue indefinitely—she reminds you that she has now been taking it consistently for 3 years. She tells you that she has continued with the same boyfriend; confident that they are in a monogamous relationship she has agreed to stop using condoms and rely on the COCP for contraception. She has been doing this for 6 months. She tells you that her boyfriend has had only one other partner and she wonders if she really needs a Pap smear. She would like more information about Pap smears generally and, in particular, wants to understand what 'HPV' infection is all about. Her last menstrual period (or more accurately withdrawal bleed) was 2 weeks previously. Kate does not smoke cigarettes.

What do you answer to Kate's questions about the 'pill'?

You explain to Kate that in the 45 years since the 'pill' has been available to Australian women there have been major changes in formulation, with current pills now containing much smaller doses of both oestrogen and progestogens. Much of the risk information about the COCP comes from research on earlier higher-dose pill types. There are three main concerns about the safety of the COCP: thromboembolic disease, cardiovascular disease and breast cancer. Although statistically Kate's chances of developing any of these are slightly raised by long-term pill taking, since she is a healthy young non-smoker taking a second-generation pill her absolute risk is extremely small for all conditions. You also briefly outline for Kate the advantages of the COCP. You point out that, as with any medication, there are always risks and benefits, and that ultimately it is her choice to make an informed decision about this medication.

Clinical comment

Numerous types of COCP have been developed and used since the 1960s:

- First generation—first prescribed in early 1960s; oestrogen as ethinyloestradiol (up to 100 µg) plus norethisterone or its derivatives.
- Second generation—oestrogen (usually 20–30 µg) plus levonorgestrel or related progestogen.
- Third generation—oestrogen plus desogestrel, norgestimate or gestodene.

- Pills containing oestrogen plus anti-androgen (e.g. cyproterone acetate or drosperidone) instead of a progestogen, are used for women with acne, mild hirsutism or other evidence of the polycystic ovarian syndrome, who may or may not also require contraception.
- Pill formulations may be monophasic (same dose of oestrogen and progesterone every day), biphasic (a two-step progestogen dose with constant oestrogen dose) or triphasic (three-step progestogen dose, two-step oestrogen dose). Triphasic pills offer no advantage over monophasic, cannot be taken in continuous regimens and are associated with more breakthrough bleeding than monophasic pills.
- COCPs are extremely effective contraceptives with a Pearl Index of 0.1. The Pearl Index is derived from the formula: Method failure rate (in number of pregnancies per 100 woman-years) = (total accidental pregnancies ×1200)/total months of exposure. (Note that the Pearl Index refers to 'method failure'; in real life 'failure' of a method may also be attributable to 'user failure'.)

Safety of the combined oral contraceptive pill

- Thromboembolic disease—there is an increased risk of venous thromboembolism in 'pill' users of about three times the risk of non-pill users. The figures are 5 cases per 100 000 in non-pill users, 15 per 100 000 in second-generation pill users and 30 per 100 000 in third-generation pill users per year. It is worth noting that the incidence in pregnant women is 300 per 100 000.
- Arterial thrombosis is more common in women with uncontrolled hypertension and/or diabetes, smokers or those with a family history. The COCP is *not* contraindicated in well-controlled hypertension or diabetes, although women with these conditions should be kept under regular observation.
- Breast cancer—use of a combined pill slightly increases the risk of breast cancer in women over the age of 40. The increase is of localised disease and may be due to the progression of pre-existing disease; some studies were done at a time when higher-dose pills were prescribed. The prognosis is good.
- There is a possible small increase in the risk of cervical cancer for users of the combined pill. The importance of regular cervical screening should be emphasised to all women. Hepatic adenoma is a rare risk of the combined pill.

As well as being an extremely reliable contraceptive method, the COCP is very effective treatment for primary dysmenorrhoea, it reduces the amount of menstrual blood loss, therefore reducing the incidence of anaemia, and allows for manipulation of cycle length. It also reduces the incidence of endometriosis, fibroids, ovarian cysts and ovarian cancer, endometrial cancer, benign breast disease and premenstrual syndrome, and offers some protection against pelvic inflammatory disease.

Contraindications to the combined oral contraceptive pill

- History of thromboembolic disease
- Existing cardiovascular or cerebrovascular disease or history of these
- Breast cancer
- Known liver disease or markedly abnormal liver function tests or jaundice
- Uncontrolled or severe hypertension
- Poorly controlled diabetes or diabetes complicated by vascular disease
- History of frequent migraine attacks
- Women over 35 years smoking more than 15 cigarettes per day
- Active gallbladder disease

Should Kate have a Pap smear?

Yes. First, you explain to Kate that human papillomavirus (HPV) infection is a common although usually transient condition in women her age around the time they become sexually active. Coming across HPV, Kate, you say, can really be seen as part of becoming sexually active. There are more than 100 subtypes of HPV. Some of these (e.g. subtypes 2, 6, 11) may actually cause visible papillomata or warts on the vulva, in the vagina, on the cervix or around the anus, but many can be present without causing visible warts. Some subtypes (especially types 16 and 18 but also others) are considered high risk for the development of premalignant change in the cervical epithelium, or less commonly the vaginal or vulval epithelium. While HPV is necessary for premalignant change we know it is not the whole story. Other factors are involved—in other words HPV is necessary but not sufficient for the development of premalignant and malignant change in the cervix. Cigarette smoking has been implicated as an associated factor and you note with approval that Kate does not smoke.

In the majority of cases, women are only temporarily infected with HPV—their own immune systems deal with the virus and it causes no further problems. In about 3% of women infected with subtypes 16, 18 and more rarely other types, dysplastic changes occur and, if undetected and untreated, may progress to a high-grade squamous intraepithelial lesion (HSIL) and eventually invasive cancer of the cervix. The estimated time for high-risk HPV infection to progress to HSIL is a minimum of 6 years.

You explain to Kate that you understand her questions but because there is the possibility of sexual transmission of HPV from her partner to herself, it is recommended that she have regular Pap smears. These may or may not show up signs of the presence of HPV, but should premalignant change develop the chances of detecting it are high. Pap smear screening, although it may detect HPV, is really about preventing the development of cervical cancer.

'Are Pap smears 100% effective at preventing cancer?'
Kate wants to know

No, you reply, but they are very effective. The cancer in question is usually cancer of the cervix, but occasionally cancer of the vagina or endometrium may be diagnosed following an abnormal Pap smear report. Pap smears are a screening test—they aim to detect changes that require further investigation leading to a positive or negative diagnosis. Since Pap smears were developed by Dr Papanicolaou in the 1920s and since Pap smear screening became widespread towards the end of the 20th century, cancer of the cervix, from being a common killer of women, has become rare in Australia and other developed countries, but we must stay vigilant—in countries where Pap smear screening is not available women still often die from cervical cancer.

You also offer Kate a chlamydia screening test as part of her well-woman check, explaining that this is your normal practice.

A Pap smear is a screening test, not a diagnostic test.

Clinical comment

Characteristics of a screening test

- The purpose of a screening test is to give a reasonable probability that the disease or condition being screened for is or is not present (sensitivity). All screening tests will have a certain proportion of false positive results (i.e. the test is positive but the condition is not present) and false negative results (i.e. the test is negative although the condition is, in fact, present) and the percentages of these should be known to those performing the tests. An ideal screening test should have a high sensitivity and low false positive rate. A negative smear result in a woman with worrying symptoms such as postcoital bleeding, intermenstrual bleeding or abnormal vaginal discharge should not be regarded as an exclusion of cancer.
- If a screening test is positive, further tests may be offered to reach a definite diagnosis (specific tests).
- A screening test should be minimally invasive, not harmful and relatively inexpensive since it is being offered to large numbers of people.
- A treatment should exist for the condition being screened for.

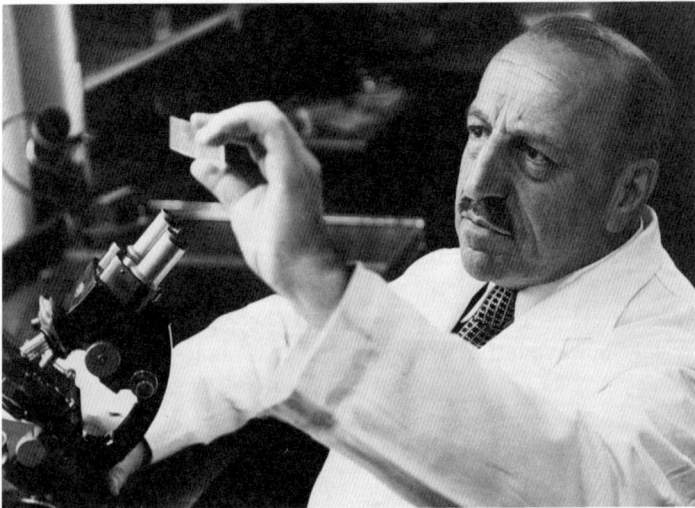

Figure 1.1 Dr Papanicolaou and his wife Mary worked at Cornell University, New York, developing the techniques of cervical screening that have led to today's national cervical screening programs.

'Should my boyfriend be tested?' Kate asks

You explain that cancer of the penis is rare. Even if Kate returns a positive smear result there is no reason for her partner to be examined unless visible warts (papillomata) are present. If this is the case these should be treated, although it is worth noting that visible warts are usually caused by low-risk HPV types.

What examination does Kate require?

You conduct a general examination of Kate, including measuring her blood pressure and examining her abdomen, then pass a vaginal speculum to inspect the cervix and take a Pap smear and a swab for chlamydia PCR testing, and perform a bimanual vaginal examination. You find that all is within normal limits. You renew her prescription for the COCP. She feels happy with this and wishes to continue. You advise her that your practice will write to her with the results of her Pap smear and chlamydia test in 2–3 weeks time and that her name will be placed on the state Pap smear register. Furthermore, your own practice will send her a reminder letter for her next Pap smear in 2 years time.

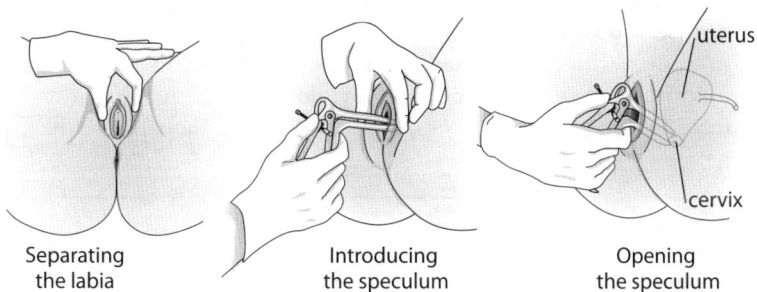

| Separating the labia | Introducing the speculum | Opening the speculum |

Figure 1.2 Taking a Pap smear

(a) The procedure of inserting a speculum to visualise the cervix. It is important to visualise the cervix and to refer the woman if an abnormality is seen, even if the Pap smear result is negative.

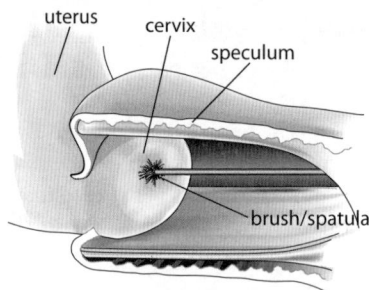

Figure 1.2 Taking a Pap smear *(cont.)*

(b) Using a brush and/or spatula, sweep through 360° at the squamocolumnar junction. Spread collected material thinly on a slide and spray with fixative before air-drying occurs, and/or place brush in transport medium for liquid-based cytology (LBC). LBC is now the normal standard of care in the United Kingdom and United States but is currently used as an adjunct in Australian practice and the cost is not covered by Medicare. In Australian practice the specimen is prepared for LBC *after* preparing the smear on the slide. With LBC, centrifuging removes debris and red cells, providing a single-layer smear for easier reading, thus resulting in fewer 'unsatisfactory' smear reports.

Cervical cytology registries (Pap smear registers) now operate in each state and territory. All information is confidential and protected by law. Women presenting for Pap smears automatically have their names included on the register unless they specifically ask not to be included ('opt out' registration). The registries sends reminders to women who are overdue for routine screening and attempt to follow up women with abnormal cytology reports for whom no record of investigation and/or treatment is known. They also provide nationwide data collection.

CP **Clinical pearls**

- Always check the whole woman—ask about concerns, take blood pressure, inquire about current contraception and plans for future pregnancy.
- Visually inspect the cervix as well as taking a Pap smear.

- Make sure that the woman knows how her Pap smear results will be communicated to her.
- Chlamydia can be screened for on a first-catch urine specimen if this is more appropriate or more acceptable to the woman concerned.

References and further reading

Dunne EF, Markowitz LE. Genital human papillomavirus infection. Clin Infect Dis 2006; 43(5):624–9.

Lenewski R, Prine L. Initiating hormonal contraception. Am Fam Physician 2006; 74(1):105–12.

National Cervical Screening Program. Australian Government Department of Health and Ageing. Available online at www.cervicalscreen.health.gov.au.

O'Connor V, Kovacs G, eds. Obstetrics, Gynaecology and Women's Health. Melbourne: Cambridge University Press, 2003:395–411, 558–60.

Shaw RW, Souter WP, Stanton SL, eds. Gynaecology. 3rd edn. London: Churchill Livingstone, 2003:583 et seq.

Society of Obstetricians and Gynecologists of Canada. Canadian Contraception Consensus Parts 1, 2 and 3. Available online at www.sogc.org.

Van Vliet H, Grimes D, Helmerhorst F, Schulz K. Biphasic versus triphasic oral contraceptives for contraception. Cochrane Database Syst Rev 2006; 3:CD003283.

Van Vliet H, Grimes DA, Helmerhorst F, Schulz K. Biphasic versus monophasic oral contraceptives for contraception. Cochrane Database Syst Rev 2006; 3:CD002032.

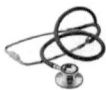

Case 2
Elena comes for a postnatal check ...

Elena is a 30-year-old woman who gave birth 4 months ago to a healthy daughter, Shona, who is currently fully breastfed. Elena commenced on the low-dose progesterone-only pill while still in the hospital after the birth of Shona. As well as returning to see you following the birth, Elena seeks contraceptive advice. Shona's birth was an uneventful spontaneous vaginal delivery and Elena's pregnancy was uncomplicated. Elena has recommenced sexual activity with her partner but reports some discomfort with intercourse; otherwise she is well and delighted with the arrival of her baby.

What further information do you need from Elena's history?

You will make general inquiries about bowel and bladder function as well as how she is coping with her baby. It is opportune to offer a Pap smear if this is due. In fact, on looking through Elena's notes you recall that at the age of 28 Elena had treatment (a loop diathermy excision of the cervix) for a high-grade epithelial abnormality (HSIL in the current nomenclature, CIN 2 in the former classification; see Table 2.1).

Elena was advised to have annual Pap smears for three years following her treatment. In fact, because of her pregnancy it is now 15 months since her last Pap smear, which was reported as negative. In that time the national recommendations for women in Elena's situation have come to include testing for high-risk HPV types until two tests are negative.

What examination do you perform for Elena?

After admiring Shona and handing her into the care of one of your practice nurses, you carry out a short general physical examination for Elena, including taking her blood pressure and an abdominal examination. The uterus has completely involuted and no masses are palpable. You proceed

Table 2.1 Comparison of terminology in Pap smear reporting

Previous terminology	Current terminology
Squamous abnormalities: atypical cells	Possible low-grade squamous intraepithelial lesion (LSIL)
Cervical intraepithelial neoplasia 1 (CIN 1)	Definite LSIL
Possible high-grade lesion, inconclusive	Possible HSIL
CIN 2	Definite HSIL
CIN 3	Definite HSIL
Glandular abnormalities: low-grade epithelial abnormality	Atypical glandular cells of undetermined significance
Low-grade epithelial abnormality	Atypical endocervical cells of undetermined significance
Inconclusive, possible high-grade glandular abnormality	Possible high-grade glandular lesion
High-grade epithelial abnormality	Endocervical adenocarcinoma-in-situ

to vaginal examination and attempt to pass a speculum but this causes marked discomfort and inspection shows the vaginal walls to be reddened and atrophic in appearance.

What is the cause of this appearance?

You explain to Elena that the low oestrogen levels that normally accompany lactation plus her use of the low-dose progesterone pill have produced a state of atrophic vaginitis, which is the cause of her dyspareunia (pain during sexual intercourse). You also explain that taking a Pap smear today may produce a scanty and unsatisfactory specimen. You recommend a small dose of topical oestrogen twice weekly, which will improve the vaginitis and reduce dyspareunia. Elena tells you that she wishes to continue breastfeeding until Shona is 6 months old, when she will be returning to work. She will continue the mini-pill, which is otherwise satisfactory, and then change to a combined oestrogen/progestogen formulation after weaning Shona. You explain that small doses of topical oestrogen will not interfere with breastfeeding or pose any risk to the baby. You arrange to see Elena in 4 weeks' time for further examination and a Pap smear.

How do you manage the following visit?

When Elena returns for this next visit she reports a great improvement in her symptoms, which she admits had been interfering somewhat with her relationship with her partner. You repeat the vaginal examination and on this occasion the vagina appears pink and 'well oestrogenised'. You take a Pap smear and a sample for HPV testing. Subsequent reports are both negative.

Elena asks you about the etonogestrel implant which she is considering as a form of contraception once she stops breastfeeding. Being so busy caring for a small baby, she remarks, 'I'm often afraid I'll forget to take the pill'. She wants to know about the implant and wonders whether vaginal dryness and discomfort is a potential problem for her if she has an implant inserted.

What is your response to her question?

The progestogen-only pill contains a small dose of oral progestogen without oestrogen. It acts by causing thickening of the cervical mucus and a thin atrophic endometrium, thereby inhibiting both sperm mobility and implantation. It has no effect on lactation (oestrogen in the combined pill may inhibit lactation) and is also useful for women in whom the COCP is contraindicated. It is highly effective, with a Pearl Index of 0.5. It is only likely to be associated with atrophic vaginitis during lactation due to the very low levels of oestrogen associated with breastfeeding.

The etonogestrel implant is a Silastic rod about the size of a matchstick that releases a steady dose of etonogestrel over a period of 3 years. (Towards the end of this time blood levels of this synthetic steroid may decline.) Etonogestrel acts by suppressing the luteinising hormone (LH) surge, so that early follicular development and oestradiol production occur without ovulation. The endometrium is thin but not atrophic; amenorrhoea results in most women but spotting and unpredictable bleeding can occur in up to 20% of women. Sufficient oestrogen is produced to avoid the symptoms of atrophic vaginitis and dyspareunia that Elena has experienced on the progestogen-only pill during lactation. The implant needs to be inserted and removed by a medical practitioner with appropriate training; occasionally when the device has been incorrectly placed surgical removal under ultrasound scanning is needed. The etonogestrel rod provides very effective contraception with a Pearl Index of 0.09 and minimal side effects, apart from the bleeding already mentioned.

You provide Elena with written material about contraceptive options to consider over the following months until she ceases breastfeeding, and make another appointment to discuss contraception with her.

Other methods of administration of progestogens for contraception include 3-monthly depot medroxyprogesterone acetate (DMPA) injections and the levonorgestrel-releasing intrauterine contraceptive device (IUCD), which has a life-span of 5 years. Both usually produce complete amenorrhoea, although spotting and light unpredictable bleeding are side effects, especially in the first few months of use. Although levels of oestradiol in the low–normal range may be observed in women using DMPA, symptoms and signs of hypo-oestrogenism, such as vaginal dryness and dyspareunia, are not a recognised side effect of either long-term method of progestogen-only administration. There is the possibility that osteoporosis may develop with long-term DMPA use—this may be assessed with serial bone mineral density measurements. Both methods are also suitable treatments for dysfunctional uterine bleeding, whether or not contraception is desired.

Clinical pearls

- Always check the whole woman as well as the pelvic organs.
- At a postnatal visit, consideration of a change of contraceptive method from that used pre-pregnancy may be appropriate.

References and further reading

Gupta S. Progestogen-only contraception: a review. Practitioner 2005; 249(1667):90–6.

National Health and Medical Research Council. National Cervical Screening Program. Screening to Prevent Cervical Cancer: Guidelines for the Management of Asymptomatic Women with Screen Detected Abnormalities. Canberra: NHMRC, June 2005.

O'Connor V, Kovacs G, eds. Obstetrics, Gynaecology and Women's Health. Melbourne: Cambridge University Press, 2003:395–411, 558–60.

Case 3
Felicity is recalled for an abnormal Pap smear report ...

Felicity is a 25-year-old woman for whom you performed a well-woman check and Pap smear some 2 weeks previously. This was the first occasion on which Felicity had presented to your practice and she told you that although she was taking the oral contraceptive pill she wanted to stop this soon to try to become pregnant. She wanted a check-up 'to make sure everything was all right down there' before she did this. It had been at least 3 years since her last Pap smear was done in a town in another state; she gave an uncertain history of a minor abnormality on a Pap smear at the age of 18 but was sure she had had normal Pap smear results since then.

Felicity's Pap smear report now reads: 'Specimen satisfactory for examination. Endocervical cells present. Severely dysplastic squamous cells present: HSIL (CIN 3)'. You have recalled her to discuss the findings, asking your receptionist to give her an early appointment and to assure her that there is no cause for alarm. Nevertheless, when Felicity arrives in your consulting room she is obviously concerned.

How do you manage Felicity's understandable anxiety?

You explain clearly to Felicity that she does not have cancer, that there are simply some changes reported in her Pap smear result that will require investigation and probably some minor surgery and follow-up. You emphasise that Pap smears are screening tests and do not supply a final diagnosis, merely an indication for further investigation. She will be wise to continue with the contraceptive pill until the investigation and any treatment is complete but she will then be able to try for a pregnancy. The treatment will not affect her ability to conceive. However, she may need to be carefully watched in a pregnancy following treatment to her cervix as there is a slightly increased risk of miscarriage or preterm labour following these cervical procedures. You take the opportunity to mention to Felicity that prior to trying to conceive she should commence on regular folic acid supplements and that screening for rubella immunity is recommended.

You then explain that HSIL is a premalignant condition that may progress to cervical cancer if left untreated.

'What kind of treatment will I have?' asks Felicity

That will depend on the treating gynaecologist, you explain. You plan to get an early appointment for Felicity at the colposcopy clinic in your local hospital. The gynaecologist will inspect the cervix using the magnification of the colposcope for closer examination and identification of possible abnormal areas and the extent of these. He or she will biopsy any abnormal areas. If histological examination of the biopsy confirms a high-grade lesion, then either laser treatment or a loop excision procedure using diathermy (large loop excision of the transformation zone [LLETZ]) will be recommended. The laser is used with local anaesthesia; LLETZ may be done with local or general anaesthesia. In both types of treatment the doctor will first inspect the cervix again with a colposcope to identify the abnormal area or areas in

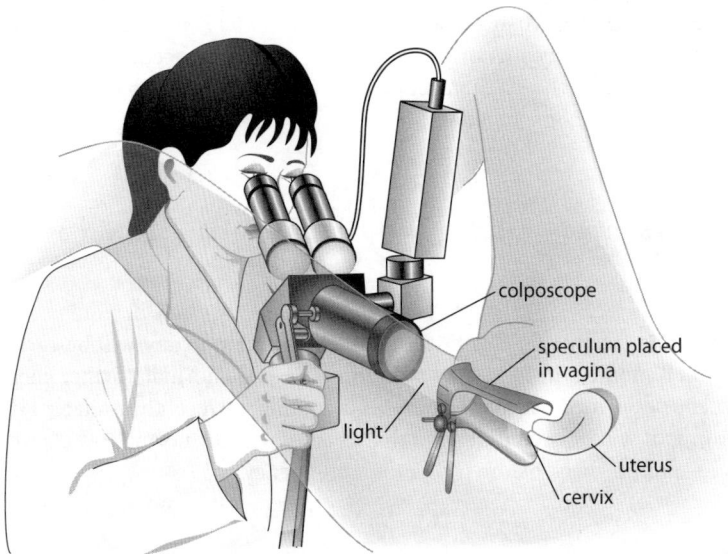

Figure 3.1 Colposcopy procedure. Through the colposcope a magnified view of the cervix is obtained. Abnormal areas are inspected and directed biopsies can be taken.

order to try to remove all abnormal tissue. Following the procedure there will be some vaginal discharge for 7–10 days.

In cases where the whole lesion cannot be visualised, the lesion is very large, there is a discrepancy between cytology and target biopsy or adenocarcinoma or microinvasive disease is suspected, a cone biopsy may be performed using a scalpel ('cold knife cone biopsy') and the cervix sutured.

'Are there any risks to these procedures?' Felicity wants to know

Rarely, there may be moderate to severe bleeding requiring return to hospital and possible diathermy or suturing of bleeding points. However, subsequent bleeding is usually mild and due to secondary infection. Such bleeding is usually treated with broad-spectrum antibiotics—oral amoxicillin or a cephalosporin and metronidazole would be a suitable combination. Serious but very rare complications include injury to adjacent organs (e.g. bladder or bowel) requiring surgical repair. Complications following cone biopsy are more frequent than those following the LLETZ procedure. Cervical stenosis causing dysmenorrhoea (painful periods) or reduced or absent periods (amenorrhoea) can occur; cervical stenosis can also interfere with the ability to become pregnant.

'When can I try to become pregnant after all this?' Felicity asks

Following treatment a further Pap smear and colposcopy will be carried out in 3 months. If the results of both of these are normal, further checks will be performed in 6 and 12 months including the recently available HPV testing. It will be recommended that Felicity wait for normal results from the 6-month check before trying for a pregnancy.

'How much will the treatment affect my chances of becoming pregnant or continuing with the pregnancy?'—Felicity specifically wants to know the answers to these questions

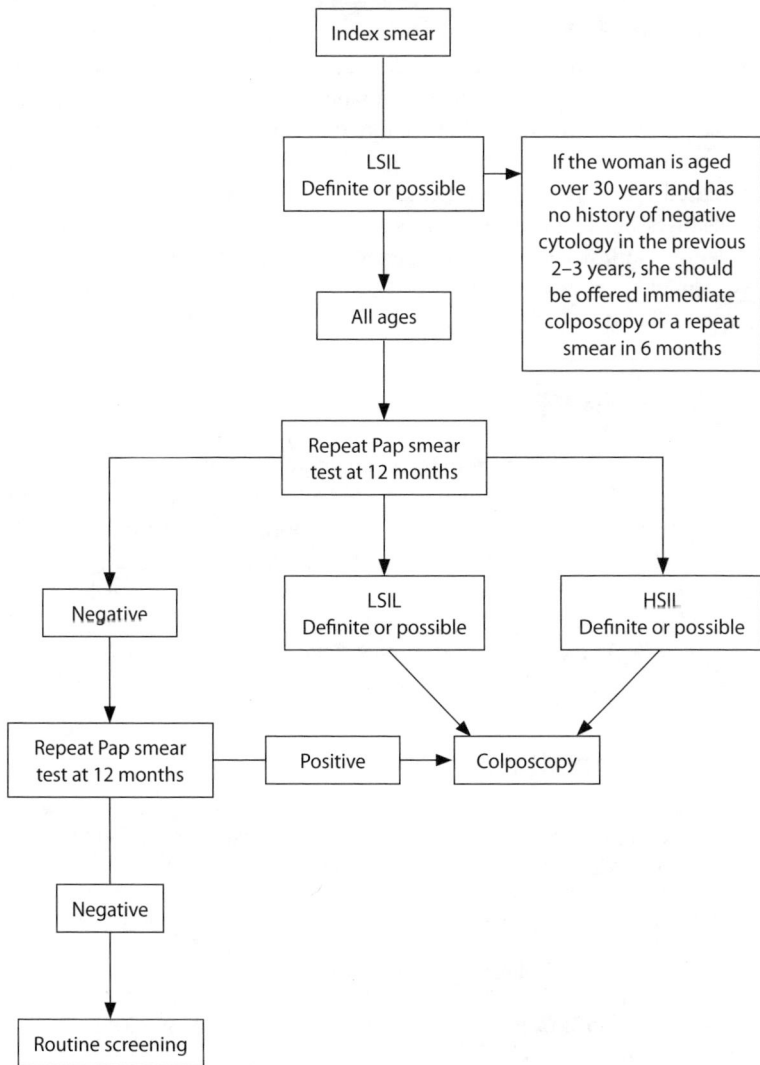

Figure 3.2 Flow chart for the management of definite or possible low-grade Pap smear reports. Note that women with possible/definite LSIL at a first smear are referred for immediate colposcopy only if aged 30 years or more and with no history of a negative smear report in the previous 2 years.

(From National Health and Medical Research Council. Screening to Prevent Cervical Cancer: Guidelines for the Management of Asymptomatic Women with Screen Detected Abnormalities. Canberra: NHMRC, June 2005)

After the surgery the cervix heals, with the formation of a new squamocolumnar junction. In most cases the cervix functions normally and there is no barrier to conception. Very occasionally as already mentioned, cervical stenosis may follow a LLETZ procedure or a cone biopsy and dilatation of the cervix may be needed. Following a LLETZ procedure there is a slightly increased incidence of miscarriage or preterm labour. Repeated LLETZ procedures or cone biopsy of the cervix may result in shortened cervical length and/or cervical incompetence. In such cases careful specialist assessment is needed and insertion of a cervical suture during pregnancy may be advised.

Clinical pearls

Each year in Australia more than 1000 new cases of cervical cancer are diagnosed and over 300 women die from the disease. With regular Pap smears and appropriate treatment when abnormalities are detected, most cervical cancer could be prevented. The development and introduction of vaccines that are protective against two common high-risk subtypes of HPV (subtypes 16 and 18) and two subtypes commonly causing genital warts (subtypes 6 and 11) offer the possibility of prevention of the majority of cervical cancers in the near future.

References and further reading

BerghellaV, Pereira L, Gariepy A et al. Prior cone biopsy: prediction of preterm birth by cervical ultrasound. Am J Obstet Gynecol. 2004 Oct;191(4):1393–7.

Finn M, Bowyer L, Carr S, O'Connor V, Vollenhoven B, eds. Women's Health— a Core Curriculum. Sydney: Elsevier, 2005:254–8.

Frazer IH, Cox J. Finding a vaccine for human papillomavirus. Lancet 2006; 367(9528):2058.

Garland SM. Human papilloma vaccines—challenges to implementation. Sex Health 2006; 3(2):63–5.

Lindeque BG. Management of cervical premalignant lesions. Best Pract Res Clin Obstet Gynaecol 2005; 19(4):545–61.

Mathevet P, Chemali E, Roy M et al. Long-term outcome of a randomized study comparing three techniques of conization: cold knife, laser, and LEEP. Eur J Obstet Gynecol Reprod Biol. 2003 Feb 10;106(2):214–8.

National Health and Medical Research Council. National Cervical Screening Program. Screening to Prevent Cervical Cancer: Guidelines for the Management of Asymptomatic Women with Screen Detected Abnormalities. Canberra: NHMRC, June 2005.

Rolling out HPV vaccines worldwide. Lancet 2006; 367(9528):2034. Editorial.

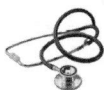

Case 4
Christine's periods are becoming heavier …

Christine is a 41-year-old nurse who attends your practice intermittently. Christine's periods have become increasingly heavy over the past few years.

What history do you take from Christine?

Christine remembers that when she last saw you for a Pap smear 4 years ago her periods were normal. She consulted you at that time for a referral for sterilisation as she had completed her family and wanted to stop taking the COCP. Laparoscopic sterilisation was performed 6 months later at the local hospital. Since then, her periods have become heavier. During the first 4–5 days of her period she passes large clots, and also has flooding, which is enough to bypass both a tampon and a large menstrual pad. She has had some accidents with blood on her clothes, which she finds mortifying. Her periods still occur regularly every 28 days, but have lengthened to 7–8 days, although the heavy bleeding is limited to the first 4–5 days. She has some pain related to passing the larger clots, but otherwise experiences only mild discomfort during menstruation. She feels tired and worn out most of the time, which she attributes to her long working hours and the pressures of having to bring up a young family. Christine is wondering whether she can be referred for a quick 'clean-out' dilatation and curettage (D&C) so her periods can go back to normal.

> Menstrual loss is usually significantly reduced with COCP use—it is possible that the COCP had effectively prevented Christine's heavy menstrual loss, which was revealed after she ceased the pill following the sterilisation. Many women blame tubal ligation as the cause of any subsequent menstrual problems.

Clinical comment

Menorrhagia

- Menorrhagia (heavy periods) is common in the later reproductive years.
- It is formally defined as blood loss greater than 80 mL per cycle, but as women do not commonly measure menstrual loss the symptom is largely subjective.
- It is best to record, in the patient's own words, the nature of her loss.
- Remember to perform a Pap smear if your patient is due, or overdue, for the next smear.
- Obtaining effective menstrual hygiene can be expensive if a woman has very heavy periods, as these products are classed as toiletries rather then medical aids.
- Dilatation and curettage is a diagnostic procedure and does not have a therapeutic effect.

What are the important points to note in your consultation with Christine?

It is important to ask whether there is any bleeding between periods, bleeding after sexual intercourse (postcoital bleeding) or whether she has any abnormal vaginal discharge. You should also ask if she has been experiencing any symptoms of menopause, such as missed periods or hot flushes.

Christine reports that she does not have any of these symptoms.

What examination do you conduct for Christine?

Firstly, you explain that you would like to examine her, including a pelvic examination and a Pap smear, as she is overdue for this test. You examine Christine's conjunctivae and nail beds to assess clinical signs of anaemia, and note that she does appear quite pale. Next, you examine her abdomen, looking for any masses, in particular to assess whether there is an enlarged uterus arising from the pelvis. Then, you perform a speculum examination and Pap smear, noting that Christine's cervix appears normal. Finally, you perform a bimanual pelvic examination to assess the size, consistency and position of her uterus, and palpate both adnexae to exclude any masses, also noting whether any part of the examination elicits pain or tenderness. You find that Christine has a normally sized anteverted uterus with no adnexal masses or tenderness.

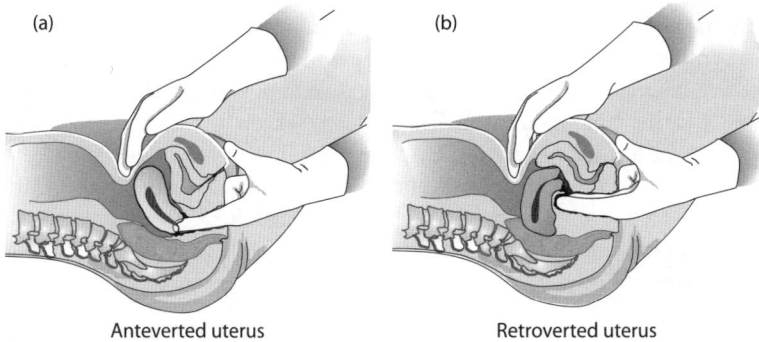

Figure 4.1 Performing a bimanual vaginal examination The uterus is palpated for size, shape and position, and the adnexae are palpated for enlargement or tenderness. **(a)** Anteverted uterus. **(b)** Retroverted uterus.

Menorrhagia—important clinical points

- Menorrhagia can result in anaemia.
- Always examine the woman fully, including blood pressure and abdominal and bimanual pelvic examination.
- If the uterus is enlarged, the diagnosis may be uterine fibromyomata (fibroids) or adenomyosis. Pelvic ultrasound may be useful in this circumstance.
- If the uterus is of normal size, pelvic ultrasound is rarely helpful.
- Malignancy (endometrial carcinoma) is rare in the premenopausal age group. One should always inquire about intermenstrual bleeding, postcoital bleeding and abnormal vaginal discharge. Referral to a gynaecologist is mandatory in these circumstances. Women over the age of 45 or obese women (who are at greater risk of endometrial cancer) may also need to be referred early for specialist opinion.

What investigations are indicated for Christine?

You arrange a full blood count (FBC) to assess the possibility of anaemia, and discuss the likely causes of the heavy bleeding with Christine. At this stage, you feel that there is no need to refer her to a gynaecologist as the periods, although heavy, are not alarming, there are no symptoms to suggest malignancy, and there are no abnormal findings on examination to suggest uterine fibroids, endometriosis or pelvic inflammatory disease. You explain to her that a D&C does not have a therapeutic effect, and will be unlikely to return her periods to normal. There are several possible treatment options for Christine, both medical and surgical. She is keen to avoid surgery as she cannot afford the time off work. You explain that common medical treatments include non-steroidal anti-inflammatory drugs (NSAIDs), tranexamic acid, the COCP and the levonorgestrel-releasing IUCD. For completeness, you also explain to her that the surgical options include endometrial ablation and hysterectomy.

Clinical comment

Medical options for the treatment of menorrhagia

- NSAIDs (e.g. mefenamic acid, naproxen) can bring about up to 50% reduction in menstrual loss. Ideally, they should be commenced 5–7 days prior to menstruation. They are also good for reducing menstrual pain. The main side effect is gastric irritation.
- Tranexamic acid, an anti-fibrinolytic, can produce up to 80% reduction in menstrual loss. It is taken only on days of heavy bleeding. The most common side effect is abdominal bloating.
- Periods are lighter and less painful on the monophasic COCP. Various types of COCP can be tried if initially unsuccessful, but they need to be continued for three cycles before the effect can be gauged. They are useful if contraception is required.
- Progestogen-releasing IUCD. This is the most effective medical therapy for menorrhagia, with a 95% reduction in menstrual loss, and it can remain in situ for 5 years. The most common complaint is daily spotting for the first 3–5 months; women should be warned in advance that this may happen. The IUCD also provides contraception for women requiring this.

Surgical options for the treatment of menorrhagia

- Endometrial ablation—50% of patients become amenorrhoeic, 40% have reduced periods and 10% are unchanged. The variety of different methods available (roller-ball, loop resection, thermal balloon, microwave, radiofrequency ablation and bipolar electrode) testify to the fact that no one procedure has yet proved its superiority. The procedure is best reserved for women in their mid–late 40s because in younger women periods tend to return over the years. It is not a

contraceptive and, if sterilisation has not been performed or is not performed concurrently, contraception must be provided.
- Hysterectomy—this may be abdominal, vaginal or laparoscopic. There is a 100% guarantee of success, but it remains major surgery with all of the associated risks. In general, it should remain the last option.

How do you follow up Christine?

Two weeks later, Christine returns to you for the results of her tests and her decision regarding treatment. Her Pap smear report is normal, and you remind her that she needs to have another one in 2 years time. You provide her with a reminder card. Her FBC shows a haemoglobin (Hb) value of 95 g/L and you place her on oral iron supplements until the treatment for reducing the degree of menstrual blood loss is successful. She has decided to try tranexamic acid because she feels this will suit her circumstances best. You arrange for her to see you again in 3 months' time, with a menstrual calendar recording her loss so you can both review the success of this approach.

Clinical pearls

- A woman with heavy but regular periods and with normal findings on general clinical examination does not require immediate gynaecological referral—medical treatment can be tried.
- Remember to ask about intermenstrual or postcoital bleeding—these symptoms, or any history of irregular bleeding, mean that the woman should be further investigated before any treatment is commenced.
- Do not overlook general health concerns and remember to take a Pap smear.

References and further reading

Duckitt K, McCully K. Menorrhagia. Clin Evid 2005; (14):2324–42.
Lethaby A, Hickey M, Garry R. Endometrial destruction techniques for heavy menstrual bleeding. Cochrane Database Syst Rev 2005; 4:CD001501.
Lethaby AE, Cooke I, Rees M. Progesterone or progestogen-releasing intrauterine systems for heavy menstrual bleeding. Cochrane Database Syst Rev 2005; 4:CD002126.

Marjoribanks J, Lethaby A, Farquhar C. Surgery versus medical therapy for heavy menstrual bleeding. Cochrane Database Syst Rev 2006; 2:CD003855.

O'Connor V, Kovacs G, eds. Obstetrics, Gynaecology and Women's Health. Melbourne: Cambridge University Press, 2003:509–17.

Osei J, Critchley H. Menorrhagia, mechanisms and targeted therapies. Curr Opin Obstet Gynecol 2005; 17(4):411–18.

Rees M, Hope S. Casebook: menorrhagia. Practitioner 2006; 250(1678):24, 26, 28–30.

Royal College of Obstetricians and Gynaecologists. National Evidence-Based Guidelines: The Initial Management of Menorrhagia. Available online at www.rcog.org.uk.

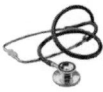

Case 5
Mai Ling is missing school because of heavy periods ...

Mai Ling is a 14-year-old schoolgirl who is brought to see you by her mother. Mai Ling has had very heavy periods for the last 12 months. She is feeling tired and listless, and is missing several days of school each month at the time of her period.

What are the important points to note in your first consultation with Mai Ling?

It is important to understand the sensitivities of dealing with a young teenager with menstrual problems. She may be embarrassed by the visit and need her mother's help in answering questions. Alternatively, she may be quite confident and may actually prefer not to have her mother present. *Note*: It is appropriate to suggest that you spend part of the consultation with Mai Ling alone. If she and her mother agree, this will give her the opportunity to raise issues of concern to her. If she indicates that she has become sexually active, you can take the opportunity to talk about effective contraception and the importance of safe sex.

You need to be sensible and circumspect when inquiring about sexual activity in a minor. There is no foolproof way to handle this question, but it is important to ask. If she is sexually active and her mother is unaware of this, you should encourage her to tell her mother but preserve patient–doctor confidentiality. This is a complex social and medicolegal situation, and advice should be sought if you think she is in any danger from her activity.

What history do you take from Mai Ling?

Mai Ling's menarche was at age 11, and for the first 12 months her periods were irregular, light and painless. About 12 months ago they became more regular, occurring once a month (indicating the onset of regular ovulation), but they have become increasingly heavy. She bleeds heavily for 7 days, regularly every 28 days, and is experiencing moderate cramping menstrual pain on day 1. She uses large pads, changed every 2 hours, on days 1–2 of bleeding. She has never used tampons. Otherwise there is no relevant medical or surgical history; Mai Ling has always been in good health.

Is there a family history of bleeding abnormalities?

Mai Ling's mother tells you there is no known history of bleeding abnormalities in the family.

What examination of Mai Ling is indicated?

You conduct a general examination of Mai Ling and specifically look for signs of anaemia. You find that she does have pale conjunctivae and is mildly tachycardic—pulse rate 90 bpm at rest. Abdominal examination reveals no masses. Mai Ling then tells you that she has never been sexually active. You explain to her that there is no reason for you to perform a vaginal examination for her.

> You should never perform a vaginal examination on a virgin. An abdominal examination is all that is required. Older authorities advocate the use of a rectal examination instead to detect any uterine masses, but we feel that this is not warranted either in a young and potentially vulnerable girl. In the rare event of abdominal palpation detecting a mass arising from the pelvis, an ultrasound scan (USS) may be performed prior to specialist referral.

What investigations do you order for Mai Ling?

Mai Ling should have an FBC performed. You also order a coagulation screen for her and testing for von Willebrand's factor.

A week later she returns to see you for the results of these tests:

- FBC: haemoglobin—90 g/L
- Coagulation screen, including testing for the absence or deficiency of von Willebrand's factor, is normal.

Bleeding diatheses must be excluded in this group of patients. von Willebrand's disease is the most common. Consider referral to a haematologist if there are blood coagulation abnormalities or a family history.

How do you now manage Mai Ling's problem?

You recommend oral iron–folate supplementation for Mai Ling, as she has iron-deficiency anaemia secondary to her excessive menstrual blood loss. You also recommend that she take a 50 μg ethynyl oestradiol COCP in order to control her heavy periods, and discuss the use of this with Mai Ling and her mother. You explain that the 'pill' has roles other than contraception. You advise her about the common initial side effects of nausea and headache, explaining that these will generally resolve quickly with continued use of the medication. You also explain that the pills may be taken continuously—for three months at a time is common practice, reducing periods to four times a year, and that this has no harmful short- or long term effects while also decreasing the amount of blood loss.

Clinical comment

Treating menorrhagia in teenagers

- Oral iron supplementation is usually only required for 2–3 months.
- In general, triphasic oral contraceptive pills are not useful for symptom control. As 30% of women still ovulate on these pills, they may not control symptoms such as menorrhagia or dysmenorrhoea. Even a 30 μg monophasic pill may not sufficiently inhibit the menstrual cycle of a teenager, and hence a 50 μg pill may be more appropriate.
- You must remember to tell the patient to take the pill every day. Missed pills will result in breakthrough bleeding or, if used for contraception, possible unplanned pregnancy.
- The COCP is also helpful in controlling menstrual pain. Other possible alternative treatments include NSAIDs and tranexamic acid, but the COCP is the easiest and most effective treatment in this age group.

When do you arrange to see Mai Ling again?

You see Mai Ling 3 months later. Her haemoglobin level is now normal and she is no longer experiencing symptoms of anaemia. Her periods now last for 3 days, and are light and pain free. They are no longer interfering with her school and sporting life. She wants to know how long she should remain on the pill. You advise her that she may continue safely on the pill until such time as she wants to have a baby but that she should return for annual check-ups with your practice. You further explain that if and when she becomes sexually active she should return to see you to make sure she completely understands the contraceptive effects of the pill and what other precautions should be taken.

Clinical pearls

- When assessing the effect of the COCP on menstrual symptoms, it is important to wait for two to three cycles to judge the outcome, as symptom control may not occur immediately. It is important not to assume therapeutic failure and change the COCP to a different variety on a monthly basis, trying to control the symptoms. This will not be effective, and can result in severe bleeding due to inappropriate hormonal manipulation.

References and further reading

Brooks MV. von Willebrand disease: an important differential for menorrhagia. Adv Nurse Pract 2006; 14(3):67–8.

Kouides PA. Current understanding of von Willebrand's disease in women—some answers, more questions. Haemophilia 2006;12 (suppl. 3):143–51.

O'Connor V, Kovacs G, eds. Obstetrics, Gynaecology and Women's Health. Melbourne: Cambridge University Press, 2003:198–201.

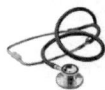

Case 6
April is bothered by acne …

April is a 16-year-old girl who comes seeking your help with acne, which has been present intermittently since she was 13 but which has become more severe in the past 6 months. She has tried various proprietary preparations with some success but is increasingly embarrassed by her skin. Her first question to you is, 'Will taking the pill help?'

What is your response to April?

You explain that you first need to know more about April and take a full history. She tells you that the acne is most marked on her face but is also present on her chest and back. She has also noticed some hair growth on her chin, uses a depilatory cream for this and is clearly embarrassed by the presence of hirsutism.

What history do you take from April?

You take a full menstrual history from April. Her periods began when she was 12. At first they were regular, 4–5 days in a 28-day cycle, but in the past year they have become unpredictable and cycles vary from 3 to 5 weeks in length and the periods themselves are sometimes light and sometimes very heavy with the passage of clots and dysmenorrhoea. On questioning, April also says that she has had a tendency to put on weight for the past 2 years, something she combats by vigorous exercise and careful attention to her diet—she is a vegetarian.

In the past April has had no serious illness or surgical operations and the only relevant family history is her mother's type 2 diabetes. She has a boyfriend but has never been sexually active, although she asks whether the 'pill' you prescribe will protect her against pregnancy if she does commence sexual activity in the future.

How do you answer this question?

You tell April that the oral contraceptive pill can certainly be very effective in preventing pregnancy but that you will want to have a full discussion with her about how it works and what precautions are necessary before prescribing it for any indication.

What examination do you perform for April?

You then conduct a physical examination for April. General examination shows a young woman of height 165 cm and weight 73 kg. She has a moderate degree of acne on her nose and cheeks and minimal hirsutism below her chin. The acne is also visible on her back and chest. Her BP is 110/70 mmHg. You inspect and palpate her abdomen—nothing abnormal is detected.

Should you perform a vaginal examination?

No. April has indicated that she is not sexually active and no useful information is likely to be gained from the examination anyway.

What is your clinical impression and what is your next step?

April's history and examination provide a diagnosis of polycystic ovarian syndrome (PCOS)—she has signs of androgen excess (acne and hirsutism), irregular menstrual cycles suggestive of unopposed oestrogen and a tendency to obesity.

PCOS is a heterogeneous disorder that may include one or more of several clinical and biochemical features. Insulin resistance is thought to be the main underlying factor; PCOS has a familial component. Resultant increased insulin production leads to increased production of ovarian androgens. Clinical features may include oligomenorrhoea, amenorrhoea, menorrhagia, infertility, obesity, and signs of androgen excess—hirsutism and acne. Biochemical abnormalities include raised serum concentrations of LH, testosterone, androstenedione, dehydroepiandrosterone sulfate (DHEAS) and insulin.

Clinical comment

Polycystic ovarian syndrome

- PCOS is the commonest hormonal disturbance affecting women.
- Polycystic ovaries demonstrated on ultrasound are present in 20–25% of women—these show hypertrophy of ovarian stroma and at least 10 follicles usually 8–10 mm in diameter arranged beneath the capsule of the ovary or less often scattered through the stroma.
- However, many women with polycystic ovaries on ultrasound do not have symptoms or signs of PCOS.

What investigations should you arrange for April?

It will be appropriate to arrange a pelvic ultrasound examination and some biochemical screening for April. She should also have an FBC performed to exclude anaemia related to heavy vaginal bleeding.

You order a pelvic ultrasound, FBC and measurements of FSH (follicle stimulating hormone), LH and androgens, and arrange to see April in 1 week's time. At this visit she is accompanied by her mother. Her mother is clearly concerned about April's condition and April is clearly embarrassed by her mother's presence.

How do you manage this situation?

You tell both mother and daughter that with April's permission you will explain the results to them both but that you would then like to see April alone and that this is your usual practice with young people of April's age.

April's ovaries show a polycystic picture (more than 10 small cystic follicles around the periphery of the ovary) but no thickening or other abnormality of the endometrium. Blood results show that LH is elevated and FSH is somewhat reduced; other hormones show normal levels, although free testosterone is in the upper normal range. You explain that April has a mild degree of a common problem and that her main concern, the acne, can be well controlled by hormonal methods or local applications. You also mention that young women with PCOS have a higher incidence of diabetes, hypertension and cardiovascular disease in later life—April's family history of diabetes is significant in this regard. You point out that attention to diet and undertaking regular exercise can have a positive impact on April's health generally and reduce the undesirable effects of PCOS.

With April alone you discuss local measures for acne and also explain that the more oestrogenic forms of the COCP, especially those also containing the anti-androgen cyproterone acetate, will regulate her menstrual cycles as well as help improve her acne. You warn her, however, that it may take several months for her to observe this improvement. You discuss the use of the COCP as a contraceptive with her in detail. She tells you that her mother will be happy with her taking the COCP for acne but that she does not wish to imply that she is contemplating sexual activity. You reassure her about patient confidentiality.

With her mother again present you prescribe a combined ethinyloestra-diol/cyproterone acetate pill to be commenced at the time of the next period and arrange to review April in 3 months time.

Clinical pearls

- Teenagers, especially older teenagers accompanied by parents, should always be offered the possibility of a consultation without parents present, and the principle of patient confidentiality should be emphasised.

References and further reading

Kovacs G, ed. Polycystic Ovary Syndrome. Melbourne: Cambridge University Press, 2000.

Moghetti P, Toscano V. Treatment of hirsutism and acne in hyperandrogenism. Best Pract Res Clin Endocrinol Metab 2006; 20(2):221–34.

Moran LJ, Brinkworth G, Noakes M, Norman RJ. Effects of lifestyle modification in polycystic ovarian syndrome. Reprod Biomed Online 2006; 12(5):569–78.

Zapanti E, Kiapekou E, Loutradis D. Treatment options of polycystic ovary syndrome in adolescence. Pediatr Endocrinol Rev 2006; 3 (suppl. 1):208–13.

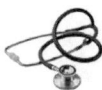

Case 7
Chloe has severe period pains ...

Chloe is a 13-year-old schoolgirl brought along by her mother to see you because of increasingly severe period pain. Each month for the past 3 months Chloe has needed 2 days away from school because of period-associated pain. This is interfering with her ability to play competition netball, which she loves. Chloe has tried paracetamol, aspirin and hot water bottles for the pain, with only partial success. Her last period, the most painful yet, has just finished.

What is the likely diagnosis here?

The most likely diagnosis is primary dysmenorrhoea due to prostaglandins produced by the disintegrating endometrium, causing painful uterine contractions. However, it is important not to overlook occasional rare causes of lower abdominal pain in young teenagers. Chloe should also be reassured so that she does not start to see her normal bodily functions in a negative light.

How do you manage this consultation?

You take a short history from Chloe, with her mother present. Her first period occurred when she was 11, and for several months cycles were irregular and periods pain-free. Over the past year her cycles have gradually become regular, with bleeding every 30 days lasting 4–5 days. Pain is cramping and begins at the same time as the bleeding, on day 1, not disappearing completely until day 3. Bleeding is not particularly heavy, by both Chloe's and her mother's estimates.

Chloe's health is otherwise good. She has occasional mild asthma but no history of allergy to any drug, including NSAIDs. She had her appendix removed at the age of 8, and her tonsils when she was 10. She is in Year 8 at school and is fitting well into school life.

Characteristically, primary dysmenorrhoea does not occur in the first cycles after the menarche, which are anovulatory, but only begins following ovulation, when the cycle usually becomes more regular. This happens 1–2 years after menarche.

What examination do you make?

You conduct a brief general physical examination of Chloe. She looks well, with no signs of anaemia, and is neither over- nor underweight. Her heart sounds are normal. Abdominal palpation reveals no tenderness or masses.

Is it necessary to perform a vaginal examination?

No. If the abdominal examination is unremarkable and with a characteristic history of primary dysmenorrhoea it can be assumed that the pelvic organs are normal. In the rare event of a lower abdominal mass being found, an ultrasound scan should be performed. You should not perform a vaginal examination in a teenager who is a virgin.

What treatment do you suggest for Chloe?

You explain to Chloe and her mother that period pain like hers is common among girls of her age but that she appears to be experiencing more pain than most. You also explain the principle of using NSAIDs in a prophylactic manner to try to prevent the dysmenorrhoea.

Prostaglandin synthetase inhibitors, by preventing the formation of prostaglandins in the endometrium, reduce future pain but are ineffective against prostaglandins already formed.

You recommend Chloe take one of the common over-the-counter NSAIDs, such as naproxen or mefenamic acid. You suggest that she keep a menstrual calendar so that she can take the NSAIDs a day before her period starts. She can continue this treatment regularly over the first 2 days of bleeding, which is when she experiences the most pain. You warn her about gastrointestinal symptoms and recommend taking the drug with food or milk.

Chloe's mother then tells you that she herself suffered painful periods for years and eventually had a hysterectomy. She is worried that Chloe may be on the same course. How do you respond?

You explain that Chloe's symptoms are quite normal and not necessarily an indication of future problems. You reinforce your approval of Chloe's already healthy lifestyle and arrange to see her in 3 months time to assess the benefits of your therapy.

Clinical pearls

- It is important when dealing with situations such as this that the girl does not come to see her normal physiology from a negative point of view.

References and further reading

Deligeoroglou E, Tsimaris P, Deliveliotou A, Christopoulos P, Creatsas G. Menstrual disorders during adolescence. Pediatr Endocrinol Rev 2006; 3 (suppl. 1):150–9.

Slap GB. Menstrual disorders in adolescence. Best Pract Res Clin Obstet Gynaecol 2003; 17(1):75–92.

Society of Obstetricians and Gynecologists of Canada: Primary Dysmenorrhea Consensus Guidelines. Available online at www.sogc.org.

Tzafettas J. Painful menstruation. Pediatr Endocrinol Rev 2006; 3 (suppl. 1):160–3.

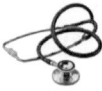

Case 8
Dorothy complains of an itch …

Dorothy is a woman of 60 who comes to see you in general practice—she has been a patient of your practice for the past 15 years.

Dorothy has always enjoyed good health and her only real problem has been with a chronic vulval itch. This first developed when Dorothy was 47, about the time she first had missed periods and occasional hot flushes. Examination at that time, according to the notes of your predecessor Dr Phillips, showed some slight vulval and vaginal atrophic changes, and he prescribed a course of topical oestrogen cream, which settled the symptoms.

A year later when Dorothy came along for her routine well-woman check she complained of continuing intermittent itch and on examination there were areas of white atrophic skin noted anteriorly on both labia majora and around the clitoris. There were no reddened or suspicious-looking areas and vaginal examination was otherwise unremarkable.

What was the clinical diagnosis here and how was the condition managed?

Dorothy was referred to a local gynaecologist who made a clinical diagnosis of lichen sclerosus but also took a small punch biopsy for histological examination, which confirmed the clinical impression. Intermittent use of either topical oestrogen or steroid cream in the form of betamethasone was recommended and for some years has kept Dorothy's symptoms under control.

What follow-up has Dorothy had?

Dorothy has had annual checks of the area ever since the initial diagnosis at your practice. There has been a gradual increase in the amount of

Lichen sclerosus is a chronic condition in which the vulval skin is pale, thickened and may be split or fissured; fusion of the labia minora and of these to the labia majora are common. The clitoris may be completely obscured by such fusion and by chronic oedema of the clitoral foreskin; dyspareunia may be a consequence. Pruritus (itch) is the most common presenting complaint. In a small number of women (up to 5%) an affected area may develop squamous cell carcinoma, hence the condition must be kept under surveillance.

skin involved and the slow development of fusion of the labia anteriorly. However, the appearances, as documented by several of your colleagues, have always been of whitened skin with no reddened areas. Dorothy has reported no dysuria or dyspareunia and has found that varying the two topical applications, together with occasional salt or Pinetarsol soaks, has kept symptoms under control. Her periods stopped completely by the age of 49, the associated menopausal symptoms were minimal and she did not wish to use any systemic hormone replacement. She has had regular Pap smears and breast checks, her blood pressure has always been in the normal range and there have been no other health problems. Dorothy does not smoke cigarettes.

Six months ago Dorothy's husband suffered a stroke and so, in fact, she has not had her usual check for more than 18 months. Today she tells you that she has noticed some slight bleeding and pain on the left side of the vulva. On examination the lichen sclerosus is evident bilaterally. On the anterior aspect of the left labium is a reddened, slightly ulcerated palpable nodule about 8 mm in diameter.

What are your concerns with this change in Dorothy's history and how do you investigate her complaint?

You complete the vaginal examination, including a cervical Pap smear. You have already performed an abdominal examination and found nothing remarkable but you now return to the abdomen and palpate the inguinal regions for enlarged lymph nodes—there are none. You tell Dorothy that you are concerned about the vulval lesion and will be arranging an early gynaecological consultation. You reassure her that although this may be an early malignancy, the fact that she has come along early, that it is small and on the skin are all good signs.

What other information may be relevant to Dorothy's situation?

You need to be aware of her home conditions as she herself may require admission to hospital. You inquire about her husband's health and find that he is recovering well. He is home from the Rehabilitation Unit and if Dorothy herself has to go to hospital her daughter will come to care for him.

The following Wednesday you receive a telephone call from the gynae-cologist, Dr Pepper. He tells you that the lesion is, in fact, a squamous cell carcinoma on biopsy, and wide local excision and excision of the left inguinal nodes has been scheduled for the following Monday with a gynaecological oncologist.

Clinical comment

Early vulval cancers are usually treated with wide local excision; dis-section of the inguinal lymph nodes is only performed if there is more than 1 mm of invasion of the primary tumour. CT scanning of the pelvis and inguinal regions may be helpful in detecting enlarged lymph nodes but has a significant false negative rate. For larger lesions, radiation and chemotherapy (using 5-fluorouracil and cisplatin) are most commonly used; they are also indicated where there are lymph node metastases. Radical vulvectomy is a very disfiguring procedure and is not now often performed.

Staging of vulval cancers uses the T (tumour), N (nodes), M (metas-tases) system: the tumour is measured and involvement of the vagina, urethra or anus, or further spread to bladder, rectum or bone is noted; groin nodes are examined postoperatively and may be free of tumour or may contain tumour on one or both sides; there may or may not be evidence of distant metastases.

What follow-up should be arranged for Dorothy?

Six weeks later Dorothy comes to see you postoperatively. She is well. Examination shows that the operation sites are well healed, although there is still some stiffness and numbness in the area. You reassure Dorothy that these symptoms will settle down and suggest gentle massage with a vitamin E cream. Dr Pepper's report states that no metastases have been detected in the lymph nodes so prognosis is good with a 90% chance of 5-year survival.

She will be attending him regularly for follow-up over the next 5 years; this will include examination of the operation site, of the lungs and abdomen and of distant lymph nodes. Lymphoedema can complicate groin node dissection.

Dorothy remarks that one thing that is now completely cured is the itch!

Clinical comment

Important points about vulval cancer

- Vulval cancer is most common in postmenopausal women but is increasing in frequency in all age groups.
- Most vulval cancers are squamous cell cancers.
- Vulval intraepithelial neoplasia—VIN I, II and III (similar to CIN nomenclature)—is a premalignant condition, but conversion to malignancy is less common and occurs more slowly than with CIN (IISIL). In some women lichen sclerosus also appears to be a premalignant condition.
- The introduction, currently in progress, of vaccines effective in protecting against four HPV subtypes (6, 11, 16, 18) will hopefully decrease the incidence of VIN and vulval cancer, as well as that of cervical cancer. Cigarette smoking should also be actively discouraged in all women and this measure should contribute to a decrease in squamous cell genital cancers.

Common causes of vulval pruritus

- Contact dermatitis due to soaps, detergents, spermicides, etc.
- Allergic dermatitis
- Drug reactions
- Infections, most commonly *Candida*
- Lichen sclerosus
- Lichen planus
- Generalised skin conditions also affecting vulva (e.g. psoriasis)
- Persistent itch and skin changes are concerning features, and the patient should be referred to a gynaecologist or dermatologist as malignancy can easily be overlooked in these patients.

CP

Clinical pearls

- Lichen sclerosus is a common condition in older women and symptoms are usually lifelong. Since up to 5% of women with lichen sclerosus may develop vulval cancer, regular inspection of the vulva should be performed annually as part of a well-woman check.

References and further reading

Gastrell FH, McConnell DT. Human papillomavirus and vulval intra-epithelial neoplasia. Best Pract Res Clin Obstet Gynaecol 2001; 15(5):769–82.

Maclean AB. Vulval cancer—prevention and screening. Best Prac Res Clin Obstet Gynaecol 2006; 20(2):379–95.

Tyring SK. Vulvar squamous cell carcinoma: guidelines for early diagnosis and treatment. Am J Obstet Gynecol 2003; 189(3 suppl.):S17–23.

Val I, Almeida G. An overview of lichen sclerosus. Clin Obstet Gynecol 2005; 48(4):808–17.

Case 9
Tammy is unexpectedly pregnant …

Tammy is a 29-year-old woman well known to your practice who comes to see you in some distress, late one Friday afternoon. Tammy has essential hypertension that has at times been difficult to control. She is currently on an angiotensin-converting enzyme (ACE) inhibitor. Tammy has two children and both pregnancies were eventful: both were complicated by severe pre-eclampsia at about 32 weeks' gestation, and the need for urgent delivery by caesarean section. Both infants required several weeks of care in the neonatal nursery and Tammy herself was in the high dependency unit for some days. The youngest child is now 12 months old. Since his birth you have had a number of conversations with Tammy and her partner Joe about contraception. Tammy understands that another pregnancy is likely to follow the same course, and she feels that her family is probably complete, but she has been reluctant to commit herself to the irreversibility of sterilisation just yet. She has also said that she does not think Joe should have a vasectomy, which he has offered to do, since 'I am the one with the health problem'.

What kinds of contraception are medically suitable for Tammy?

Tammy understands that with her hypertension she is not a suitable candidate for the COCP and she has decided against an IUCD. Prior to her second pregnancy she had 3-monthly injections of DMPA and since the birth of her second child has been taking the progestogen-only pill. Recently, she has had several sleepless nights with both her children ill, has forgotten to take the pill regularly, and the result is a positive home pregnancy test.

How do you deal initially with Tammy's presentation?

You ask Tammy how she herself feels about the pregnancy. Tammy tells you that she and Joe have been discussing the situation for 3 days now. Joe will go along with what Tammy wants to do, but he is worried about her health and the possible ill effects of another pregnancy. Tammy herself has realised that she does not want to go through another pregnancy complicated by severe pre-eclampsia, with risks to herself and the child. She is aware of the needs of her two existing children and feels she is incapable of properly caring for a third child. Tammy is requesting termination of the pregnancy and sterilisation.

Despite the lateness of the hour you take time to look at the possible options with Tammy. You outline the various scenarios, which Tammy and Joe have already considered themselves. She can be referred for excellent antenatal care in the local hospital and assisted with the care of her existing children throughout the pregnancy. However, Tammy feels that she must consider the needs of her other children, and of her partner, first. She is also aware of the teratogenic effects of ACE inhibitors in later pregnancy. She asks to be referred back to the specialist obstetrician and gynaecologist who cared for her during her pregnancies with a view to both termination and sterilisation. She asks whether the two procedures can be done under the same anaesthetic.

What is your response, and how do you advise Tammy?

You agree that this can be done. Tammy must be sure that she will not change her mind in future even should something befall one or both of her existing children or Joe. Certainly, reversal of sterilisation can be performed. Sterilisation reversal has a success rate of up to 90% in terms of successful full-term pregnancies when the sterilisation has been carried out using clips; however, it is major surgery requiring laparotomy or laparoscopy, so sterilisation must be regarded as irreversible. Tammy also needs to understand that sterilisation (Fig. 9.1) does not carry a 100% guarantee of prevention of pregnancy—about 1 woman in 1000 will become pregnant following laparoscopic clip sterilisation (figures from studies vary, and some report higher pregnancy rates). Ectopic pregnancies are more common following sterilisation.

Does Tammy meet the legal requirements for induced abortion?

Tammy meets the legal requirements for abortion in all states and territories in Australia since continuing the pregnancy clearly carries a serious risk to Tammy's physical health. Tammy's last menstrual period was about 6 weeks ago. You discuss with Tammy the possibility that she may feel upset about

a

b

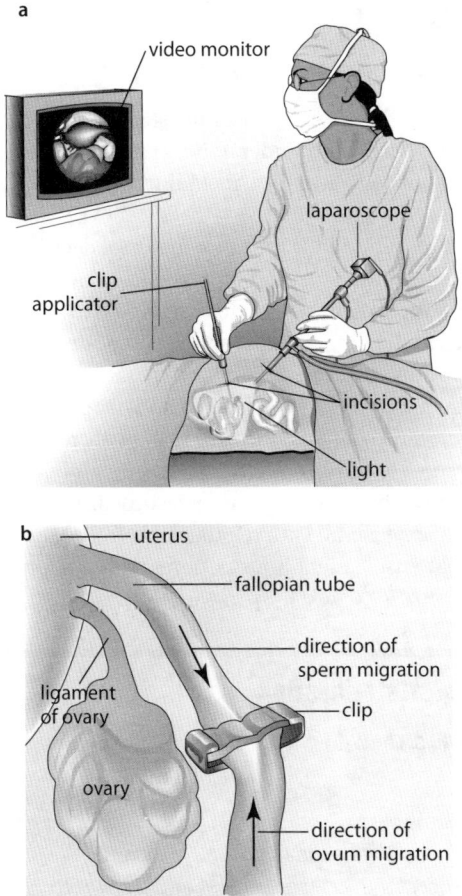

Figure 9.1 Laparoscopic sterilisation: **(a)** overview; **(b)** close-up showing how clip occludes tube

terminating the pregnancy. She acknowledges that this is so but states that she feels she is making the right decision for herself and her family. You mention that she will need a general anaesthetic for the combined procedure and that there are small but definite risks with both laparoscopy and suction curettage of the uterus. These risks include anaesthetic complications, haemorrhage, infection, damage to abdominal organs and thromboembolism. Laparotomy may need to be performed if it is not possible to perform the sterilisation laparoscopically or in the rare case of organ damage occurring. Tammy needs to be aware of all these risks before she consents to the procedures.

Clinical comment

Points for counselling prior to sterilisation

- Permanence and irreversibility of the sterilisation procedure must be clearly explained and understood.
- Other forms of contraception, including vasectomy, should be discussed.
- Time must be allowed for reflection before a decision is made.
- The failure rate of the method of sterilisation must be explained and recorded in the patient notes (this varies from 1 in 1000 women immediately following laparoscopic sterilisation to 1 in 200 women when performed in conjunction with caesarean section).
- Not infrequently, even after a detailed and unambiguous explanation and advice, women assume that this is an easily reversible procedure with full return to fertility. A clear explanation is essential, and the discussion must be comprehensively recorded. The costs of reversal of sterilisation are generally not reimbursable from Medicare.
- It is helpful to use patient information sheets and procedure-specific consent forms.

Risks of surgical sterilisation

General (i.e. can occur with any surgery)

- Chest infection
- Thromboembolism
- Cardiac arrest, stroke, death
- Risks are greater in obese patients and smokers

Specific risks of laparoscopy

- Infection—urinary tract, incision site
- Bleeding—can be severe and life-threatening if damage to major blood vessels occurs
- Damage to other organs—bladder, ureter, bowel, blood vessels
- Laparotomy may be required if there is visceral or vascular damage
- Blood transfusion may be required
- Wound hernias and scarring
- Carbon dioxide embolism is a rare and potentially fatal complication of laparoscopy
- Failure rate of all methods of tubal sterilisation

Clinical comment

Techniques of early abortion

- Early medical abortion (up to 9 weeks' gestation) has only a limited availability in Australia at the time of writing. Oral mifepristone, which may be soon more widely available in Australia, or methotrexate by injection or orally, may be given under direct medical supervision, followed by misoprostol intravaginally 1–7 days later. These various regimens result in expulsion of the products of conception in up to 98% of cases and the process can take place in the woman's home provided she has adequate support and access to 24-hour emergency care if needed. Complications include heavy bleeding, infection, and incomplete expulsion of the pregnancy with the need for surgical evacuation in about 2% of cases.
- Surgical abortion is usually by suction curettage using general or local anaesthesia and may be safely performed in a hospital or clinic in women up to 13–14 weeks of pregnancy; it can be performed later in pregnancy but risks increase with increasing gestation. Risks include uterine perforation, haemorrhage and infection.

Clinical pearls

- Surgical tubal sterilisation is generally easy to perform but less easy to reverse. Make sure that women are well informed and have time to consider the alternatives before they consent to sterilisation.

References and further reading

Dirubbo NE. Counsel your patients about contraceptive options. Nurse Pract 2006; 31(4):40–4.

Grimes DA, Creinin MD. Induced abortion—an overview for internists. Ann Intern Med 2004; 140(8):620–6.

O'Connor V, Kovacs G, eds. Obstetrics, Gynaecology and Women's Health. Melbourne: Cambridge University Press, 2003:411–14.

Peterson HB, Curtis KM. Clinical practice. Long-acting methods of contraception. N Engl J Med 2005; 353(20):2169–75.

Peterson HB, Xia Z, Hughes JM et al. The risk of pregnancy after tubal sterilization: findings from the US Collaborative Review of Sterilization. Am J Obstet Gynecol 1996; 174(4):1161–70.

Case 10
Lara is followed through a normal pregnancy ...

Lara, a 26-year-old woman, makes an appointment to see you. She reports happily that it is 7 weeks since her last menstrual period and a home pregnancy test is positive. She wants to know about options for antenatal care and delivery.

What do you tell Lara?

You congratulate Lara and ask her if she is well. She responds that she has had some slight nausea in the mornings but has no other problems. You tell her that where she chooses to book for the birth will be somewhat determined by her general health and the progress of the pregnancy, as well

---

Options for antenatal care and place of birth

- All care from a private obstetrician or general practitioner/ obstetrician and delivery by that doctor either in a private hospital or as a private patient in a public hospital.
- All care in the maternity unit of a public hospital and delivery in the birth suite of that hospital. Care may be shared with midwives if the woman is considered low risk; care in clinics and intrapartum may be from doctors at junior, registrar or specialist level depending on the complexity of the case.
- Care by public hospital midwives and delivery in a birth centre within the hospital or in a freestanding birth centre adjacent to the main hospital, with the possibility of transfer to the conventional birth suite if problems arise.
- Shared care between public hospital and general practitioners— usually for women who are low or medium risk.
- Care from an independent midwife with planned home birth.

as by whether she is in a private medical fund, but that one or more options are available locally.

Lara has no private medical cover and elects to have shared antenatal care between your practice and the local public hospital.

What history do you take from Lara?

You take a full history from Lara commencing with the date of her last menstrual period (LMP) and cycle details. Her LMP is, in fact, a withdrawal bleed following discontinuing the COCP, which she has been taking for the previous 6 years. You calculate a tentative expected date of delivery (EDD) based on the menstrual information.

> Naegele's rule: add nine months and seven days to the LMP of a woman who is certain of her menstrual dates and has regular 28-day cycles. Appropriate adjustments must be made for shorter or longer cycles.

Apart from an appendicectomy at age 15 Lara has no relevant medical, surgical or gynaecological history. She has never been pregnant before and has never had a sexually transmitted infection. She takes folic acid 0.5 mg daily but no other medications and has no allergies. Her last Pap smear 8 months previously was reported as negative.

What other history is relevant to Lara's pregnancy?

A family and a social history should be taken from all women. Lara tells you that her father has diabetes, a condition he developed at age 46. Her two younger sisters are non-identical twins. There is no history of other familial conditions or congenital anomalies that she is aware of. Lara is in a stable relationship and her partner Russell is thrilled about the pregnancy. Both partners work in banking. Lara plans to stop working at 34 weeks of pregnancy, all being well, and take 1 year's unpaid maternity leave.

What examination do you conduct for Lara?

You carry out a full general examination for her, including blood pressure, checks of the cardiovascular and respiratory systems, inspection of the breasts to note any inversion of the nipples or other condition that may interfere with breastfeeding, and examination of the thyroid gland, abdomen and lower limbs.

Does Lara need a vaginal examination?

Lara has had a well-woman check 8 months previously and has a negative Pap smear report. She does not need a repeat vaginal examination performed; however, it would be wise to arrange an ultrasound scan in the first few weeks of pregnancy since she conceived immediately after stopping the COCP and because of her close family history of multiple pregnancy. A scan performed at this gestation will give a very accurate estimation of the EDD. Transvaginal scans (TVUSS) are more accurate than abdominal scans.

> Up to 10 weeks' gestation the USS measurement (crown–rump length [CRL] of the fetus) is accurate to ±5 days. At 10–14 weeks, accuracy (of CRL or of biparietal diameter [BPD] of the head) is ±7 days. At 14–20 weeks, accuracy is ±10 days and at more than 20 weeks it is ±14 days. The most accurate USS measurement for the assessment of gestation in the second trimester is the BPD; in the third trimester it is the femur length (FL). USS dating is most accurate in the first 10 weeks of pregnancy.

You order a TVUSS for estimation of the EDD. This is performed 3 days later and confirms that Lara is pregnant—the CRL of the fetus is the mean for 7 weeks and 5 days and only one fetus is present.

What other tests should be ordered or offered to Lara in the first trimester?

Lara should have the full panel of routine antenatal blood and urine tests performed. These should be outlined to her by you before they are ordered. You should also inform Lara about screening tests for Down syndrome in the first trimester.

When should Lara be booked in for hospital delivery?

Most hospitals with shared care arrangements will wish to see Lara as early in the pregnancy as possible in order to confirm that she is suitable for

Antenatal panel of tests

- Full blood count (FBC)
- Blood group and Rh group
- Antibody screen
- Rubella antibody screen
- Hepatitis B and C screening, human immunodeficiency virus (HIV) screening—not universally practised
- Rapid plasma reagin (RPR), Venereal Disease Research Laboratories (VDRL) or other syphilis screening
- Midstream urine (MSU)
- First catch urine for polymerase chain reaction (PCR) (chlamydia and gonorrhoea)—not universal
- Endocervical swabs—not universal
- Ferritin levels, screening for haemoglobinopathies and vitamin D measurement (in women with reduced exposure to sunlight) may be appropriate in certain populations in Australia

shared care (low risk or with a medical/obstetric condition manageable in general practice) and to inform her about antenatal classes and other services provided in preparation for childbirth. The hospital will then keep records of all tests performed for Lara and a shared care card (or 'patient hand-held record') will be used to record all information derived as the pregnancy continues. Lara will be given this card to carry with her and take to all medical consultations during her pregnancy.

You arrange all routine tests and refer Lara for booking to the local hospital. You also offer Laura non-invasive screening for Down syndrome (see pp 70 and 170).

Lara returns to see you at 13 weeks' gestation. She has booked into the hospital, and is scheduled to commence antenatal classes with her partner at 20 weeks of pregnancy. Her morning sickness has settled down and she is having no difficulty coping with work.

What examination do you carry out for Lara at this and subsequent antenatal visits?

At each visit, after inquiring about Lara's general wellbeing and any specific concerns, she should have her blood pressure checked, the abdomen examined, the fetal heart listened for and a check made for oedema of the lower limbs. Urine should be tested for protein only if the blood pressure is raised. From 18 weeks onwards the presence of fetal movements should be asked about.

The abdomen should be visually inspected for the size and overall shape of the pregnant uterus in the latter part of pregnancy. From approximately 28 weeks onwards it is possible to feel fetal parts and usually to determine the lie and presentation of the baby (Fig. 10.1). From 36 weeks onwards the descent of the head into the pelvis (measured in fifths above the pelvic brim) becomes increasingly relevant (Fig. 10.2).

Abdominal palpation in pregnancy

- Fundal height—measured from the top of the pubic symphysis to the top of the uterine fundus—after 20 weeks' gestation this measurement (in cm) corresponds approximately to the number of weeks' gestation
- Lie—the relationship of the long axis of the baby to the long axis of the uterus; may be longitudinal, transverse or oblique
- Presentation—the part of the baby occupying the lower part of the uterus; usually the head (cephalic presentation), less commonly the buttocks and/or feet (breech presentation) and rarely the shoulder or an arm (in cases of transverse lie)

Visits are, by convention, 4–6 weekly to 32 weeks, 2–3 weekly to 36 weeks and weekly until delivery, although this may be modified to suit the circumstances. Some hospitals wish to see shared care patients for a further visit in the third trimester and all will require a hospital visit if a woman has passed 41 weeks' gestation.

What further tests will you perform for Lara?

Lara should also be offered a fetal morphology ultrasound scan at 18–20 weeks of pregnancy. Since she has a family history of diabetes, glucose tolerance testing should be performed at 24–28 weeks. Many centres offer routine glucose tolerance screening to all pregnant women.

Lara's blood group is A Rhesus positive and her antibody screen is negative. This screen should be repeated at 26–28 weeks. If Lara were Rhesus negative, she would have antibody screening at 28 weeks and be offered anti-D prophylaxis at 28 and 34 weeks. At 36 weeks she will have an FBC performed; in areas where syphilis is prevalent RPR may be repeated at this time. Routine screening for group B *Streptococcus* (by means of urine testing, vaginal or rectal swabs) varies from one centre to another. No other tests are indicated if Lara's pregnancy progresses otherwise uneventfully to term.

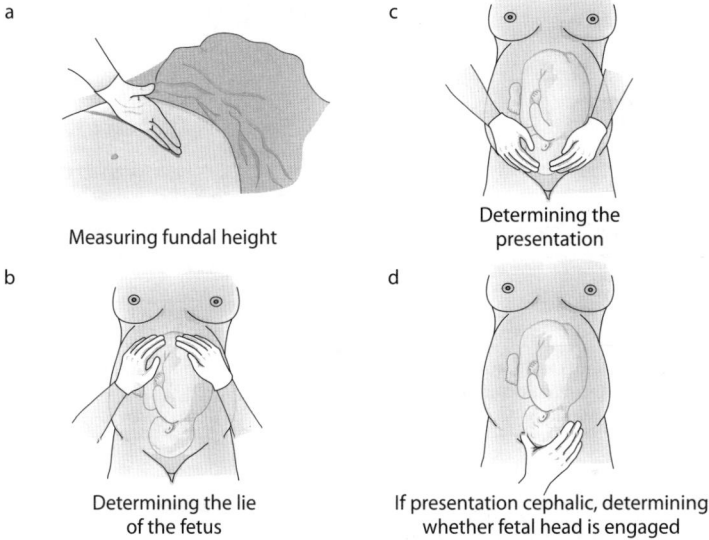

a

Measuring fundal height

c

Determining the
presentation

b

Determining the lie
of the fetus

d

If presentation cephalic, determining
whether fetal head is engaged

Figure 10.1 Palpation of the pregnant abdomen: **(a)** measuring fundal height; **(b)** determining the lie of the fetus; **(c)** determining the presentation; **(d)** when the presentation is cephalic, determining whether the fetal head is engaged

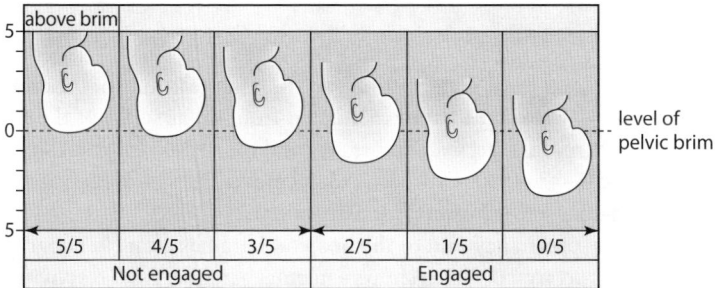

above brim

5 —

0 —

5 —

| 5/5 | 4/5 | 3/5 | 2/5 | 1/5 | 0/5 |

| Not engaged | Engaged |

level of
pelvic brim

Figure 10.2 Determination of the descent of the fetal head in a cephalic presentation. The measurement of the head in 'fifths' is demonstrated. Once three-fifths of the fetal head has passed into the pelvis, the head is termed 'engaged'.

Table 10.1 Anti-D prophylaxis for Rhesus negative women in pregnancy

Weeks	Anti-D dose (IU)
For each sensitising event[a]	
1–12	
Singleton pregnancy	250
Multiple pregnancy	625
>12	625
Postpartum	625
Routine prophylaxis[b]	
28	625
34	625

(a) Sensitising events include, for example, normal delivery, ectopic pregnancy, miscarriage, termination of pregnancy.
(b) The doses at 28 and 34 weeks are given in addition to any doses given for sensitising events.

Lara's pregnancy progresses uneventfully to 41 weeks. At this visit all observations are within normal limits. Lara, however, is anxious that she has not yet had any signs of impending labour and she feels that fetal movements have decreased in frequency over the past 24 hours.

'How long must we wait?' she asks

You explain that there is great natural variation in the timing of the onset of labour. Past 42 weeks' gestation (calculated from the first day of the LMP) there is an increase in perinatal mortality and morbidity. It is usual to offer induction at 41–42 weeks. However, as fetal movements have decreased you are referring her to the hospital for assessment.

In the day pregnancy unit of the hospital Lara has a cardiotocographic (CTG) trace performed, which shows a normal baseline, good reactivity and variability and no decelerations. She also has ultrasonic measurement of the amniotic fluid index (AFI) to assess the amount of liquor surrounding the baby; this is within the normal range. She is asked to return in 2 days' time for a further CTG; however, that evening she commences spontaneously in labour and proceeds to the uncomplicated birth of a healthy girl.

In cases of prolonged pregnancy it is usual to provide some assessment of fetal wellbeing in the 41st week, usually CTGs plus AFI at 2–3 day intervals, in addition to the usual antenatal visit.

Clinical pearls

- Maternal satisfaction with antenatal and intrapartum care is greatest when women themselves feel that they have been well informed about their options and have been active participants in decisions about their care.

References and further reading

Brown HC, Smith HJ. Giving women their own case notes to carry during pregnancy. Cochrane Database Syst Rev 2006; 3:CD002856.

Chamberlain G, Steer P, eds. Turnbull's Obstetrics. 3rd edn. London: Churchill Livingstone, 2001:105–17.

Gregory KD, Johnson CT, Johnson TR. The content of prenatal care. Update 2005. Womens Health Issues 2006; 16(4):198–215.

O'Connor V, Kovacs G, eds. Obstetrics, Gynaecology and Women's Health. Melbourne: Cambridge University Press, 2003:210–40.

Villar J, Carroli G, Khan-Neelofur D, Piaggio G, Gülmezoglu M. Patterns of routine antenatal care for low-risk pregnancy. Cochrane Database Syst Rev 2006; 3:CD000934.

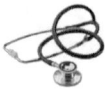

Case 11
Diane has diabetes and wants to have a baby …

Diane is a 27-year-old woman who has had Type 1 diabetes since the age of 11. She has been a patient of your general practice for her entire life. You can see from the voluminous case notes that although she had some episodes of poor sugar control in the first years of diagnosis, and was a little rebellious about her need for insulin in her teenage years, she has been well controlled for the past 9 years. Diane married 2 years ago and she is currently taking the COCP. She comes to see you today to ask about planning a pregnancy. She is aware that her diabetes poses particular problems for women like herself.

What are the initial points to be established in your discussion with Diane?

You have a short chat with Diane to confirm that her diabetes is well controlled. You find that she does regular checks with her home glucometer. She measures her blood sugar levels up to four times daily and adjusts her insulin regimen when necessary over the telephone with the local diabetes centre. Her control is generally good and her glycosylated haemoglobin (HbA_{1c}) is within the normal range. She has regular ophthalmology check-ups, and her endocrinologist reports that she has no evidence of renal disease or hypertension.

> Diane asks you, '*What are the risks of pregnancy for me and my baby?*'

As she herself has no evidence of significant diabetic vasculopathy, pregnancy will not have an adverse effect on her health. If blood glucose levels are not well controlled in early pregnancy, fetal abnormalities can occur—the risk is approximately double that of the background risk of 2–3%. Poor control later in pregnancy can lead to the fetus developing macrosomia and there is an increased risk of stillbirth. Macrosomia does not simply mean the baby is large. These babies have an abnormal distribution of fat over the upper body, and the fetal hyperinsulinaemia causing the syndrome may result in metabolic dysfunction, leading to stillbirth.

> **Pregnancy in a diabetic woman can have an adverse effect on maternal health if there is pre-existing renal impairment, hypertension secondary to renal disease or severe retinopathy. Blindness or renal failure requiring dialysis may result from continuing the pregnancy. Termination of pregnancy must be discussed in such cases.**

Diane then asks, *'Is there any way to reduce the risks to my baby?'*

You emphasise the need for good sugar control both before and after conception, and suggest that Diane also visit her endocrinologist prior to attempting to conceive as he may wish to alter her insulin regimen. You arrange for her to have a FBC, and rubella and varicella antibody screening. You recommend that Diane take folic acid 5 mg daily from now until at least the end of the first trimester. You also explain the need to report back early once she thinks she may be pregnant so that the pregnancy can be confirmed.

An early first trimester ultrasound scan for very accurate dates is important in diabetic pregnancies. Non-invasive screening for Down syndrome and related abnormalities should be offered at 10–13 weeks (see pp 70 and 170). A further ultrasound scan at 18 weeks, preferably in a fetal maternal medicine unit (tertiary scan) is required to detect fetal anomalies. A second tertiary scan at 22–24 weeks is often advised to assess fetal cardiac anatomy. Cardiac anomalies represent about 50% of all abnormalities in pregnancies in diabetic women, and these are more easily demonstrated at this gestation compared to an 18-week scan. You explain that in the event of a severe fetal abnormality being detected before 20 weeks of pregnancy, termination of the pregnancy can be offered.

Common fetal abnormalities associated with diabetes

- Neural tube defects
- Cardiac abnormalities
- Bowel abnormalities
- Urinary tract abnormalities
- Sacral agenesis

What do you need to explain to Diane about her care in later pregnancy?

As well as careful control of blood sugar levels, Diane will have regular fetal growth scans from 24 weeks, looking for evidence of macrosomia, in particular, a disproportionate abdominal circumference growth rate, and polyhydramnios.

Fetal macrosomia is associated with shoulder dystocia during vaginal delivery and an increased incidence of caesarean section for obstructed labour due to fetal size and 'macrosomic' morphology. Fetal death in utero (and subsequent stillbirth) is associated with poor control of blood glucose levels and fluctuating fetal insulin levels in the final weeks of pregnancy.

The infants of diabetic mothers are prone to hypoglycaemia, respiratory distress syndrome, polycythaemia and neonatal jaundice, hypocalcaemia and hypomagnesaemia. However, you emphasise to Diane that with good sugar control and obstetric and paediatric care she can expect to have a live and healthy baby.

Clinical pearls

- The key to a successful outcome to pregnancy in a diabetic woman lies in tight control of blood sugar levels before and throughout the pregnancy. Care should always involve a team approach, with close cooperation between obstetricians, endocrinologists, diabetes educators and paediatricians.

References and further reading

Creasy R, Resnik R, eds. Maternal–Fetal Medicine—Principles and Practice. 5th edn. Philadelphia: WB Saunders, 2004.

Cundy T. Why do poor outcomes persist in diabetic pregnancy? BMJ 2006; 333(7562):304.

Farrar D. Pre-conception care and diabetes. Pract Midwife 2005; 8(10):14, 16–18, 964–990.

Hofmanova I. Pre-conception care and support for women with diabetes. Br J Nurs 2006; 15(2):90–4.

Macfarlane A, Tufnell D. Diabetes and pregnancy. BMJ 2006; 333(7560):157–8.

McElduff A, Cheung NW, McIntyre HD et al. The Australian Diabetes in Pregnancy Society Consensus guidelines for the management of type 1 and type 2 diabetes in relation to pregnancy. Med J Aust 2005; 183(7):373–7.

Yang J, Cummings E, O'Connell C et al. Fetal and neonatal outcomes of diabetic pregnancies. Obstet Gynecol 2006; 108(3 Pt 1):644–50.

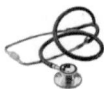

Case 12
Maria has a twin pregnancy ...

Maria is a 38-year-old woman who comes to consult you in general practice. Maria is pregnant for the fifth time. She has had four uncomplicated pregnancies resulting in the spontaneous vaginal births of four healthy sons aged 16, 14, 12 and 9. Maria and her husband have used the ovulation method of natural family planning for the past 9 years with no problems. She keeps accurate menstrual records and tells you that she has had no bleeding since her last period 8 weeks previously and is quite sure that she is pregnant. This pregnancy was unplanned but the couple are now happy with the idea of a fifth child. Maria, however, tells you that she is experiencing much more marked symptoms of early pregnancy than she remembers from her other pregnancies. She feels nauseated and exhausted for much of the day. She is suffering from heartburn, urinary frequency and nocturia, and thinks she is putting on weight very rapidly.

What further history do you need from Maria?

You need to be aware of any intercurrent medical problems Maria may have. In fact, she has been a patient of your practice for 20 years and from her notes you see that her past medical history is unremarkable. Her Pap smears are up to date.

What examination do you make for Maria?

You organise a urine beta-human chorionic gonadotrophin (β-HCG) test to confirm the pregnancy and then conduct a short general examination. Maria's BP is 120/70 mmHg, and general examination reveals no unexpected abnormality. Palpation of her lower abdomen, however, reveals a central mass arising from the pelvis and reaching to 4 cm above the pubic symphysis. After informing Maria that you think her uterus is larger than expected you use your small portable ultrasound machine to perform a transabdominal scan and have no difficulty demonstrating to

Maria two distinct pregnancy sacs with two viable fetuses, each with a CRL corresponding to 8 weeks' gestation, and two fetal hearts. Maria has a twin pregnancy.

> The causes of the finding of a 'large-for-dates' uterus on examination include wrong dates, multiple pregnancy, molar pregnancy and the coexistence of uterine pathology, such as fibroids, with normal singleton pregnancy.

While understandably Maria is somewhat overwhelmed by this news she tells you that she is quite happy about it and feels her family will be too. There is no family history of twins that she is aware of.

'Are they identical?' she asks

You explain that the presence of two separate sacs means the twins are most likely non-identical—statistically and because of Maria's age this is also more likely.

> Dizygotic twins (conception occurring with two ova released in the same cycle, and two sperm) are more common in older women and in association with in-vitro fertilisation (IVF) treatment. Dizygotic twins will each have a chorion and an amnion surrounding the developing embryo. Monozygotic twins occur when a single fertilised egg separates into two embryos: if this occurs between days 1–3 after conception each embryo develops a separate amnion and chorion; between 4–7 days there will be a single chorion but separate amnions; after day 7 twins will be monochorionic and monoamniotic. Monozygotic twins have poorer outcomes than dizygotic twins, with greater rates of early pregnancy loss, preterm delivery and perinatal mortality and morbidity.

'How will this pregnancy be different from the others?' Maria asks, *'And how will the babies be delivered?'*

'It's quite a while since I had a baby', she points out. 'After four boys, we'd love a girl but our main concern would be that the babies are healthy.'

Given her age, her parity and the fact of the twin pregnancy, you recommend that Maria have all her care in the hospital antenatal clinic. You also explain that at the age of 38 Maria has an increased risk of a fetus with Down syndrome (Table 12.1). There are screening tests and diagnostic tests for Down syndrome but with a twin pregnancy such tests can be problematic. Measurement of fetal nuchal translucency (FNT), the thickness of the skin fold at the back of the neck, can be done on each twin, with a sensitivity of 80%, but combined nuchal screening and biochemical markers (free β subunit of HCG and pregnancy-associated plasma protein [PAPP-A]) is less useful in multiple pregnancy as each twin contributes to the overall levels. Reference tables exist for twin pregnancies, but these are less accurate than for singleton pregnancies. Amniocentesis can be done for each twin under strict ultrasound control, at 15–16 weeks' gestation, or for one twin if the pregnancy is known to be monozygotic. Chorion villous sampling (CVS) can also be performed, for one fetus if they are monozygotic or both if they are dizygotic, however, there can be difficulty ensuring that separate specimens are obtained from each twin. Miscarriage rates for both CVS and amniocentesis are higher for twin pregnancies compared to singleton pregnancies. You further explain that if Down syndrome were diagnosed, termination of one or both pregnancies is an option, but that making such a decision can be extremely stressful for parents. Maria should also have an 18-week morphology scan to check for any fetal abnormalities.

Maria tells you that she will discuss this with her husband—while their religion is opposed to abortion, and she herself has always felt negative about the procedure, she is certain she would not be able to cope with twins with Down syndrome. She thinks she will probably decide to have FNT done as it is non-invasive and a negative result would give her a measure of reassurance.

What other information do you give Maria about the earlier part of her pregnancy?

You tell Maria that generally everything that can occur in a singleton pregnancy is more pronounced with twins. 'Great!' she answers. She had been about to change from a part- to a full-time teaching job. Now you suggest that she stay with part-time work and consider stopping altogether at about 28–30 weeks' gestation. The good news, you tell her, is that since she is already 8 weeks pregnant and both fetal hearts are visible it is likely that the pregnancy

Table 12.1 Age-related risks of Down syndrome

Mother's age at time of delivery (years)	Approximate risk of Down syndrome
32	1 in 660
35	1 in 355
36	1 in 300
37	1 in 220
38	1 in 165
39	1 in 125
40	1 in 90
41	1 in 70
42	1 in 50
43	1 in 40

will continue; miscarriage or loss of one twin is unlikely at this stage. You reassure her that vaginal birth is a good possibility, although there is a risk of needing a caesarean section under certain circumstances. Her morning sickness should improve after 12 weeks' gestation. Meanwhile, she should eat small, regular meals and take an iron–folate preparation.

Clinical comment

The minor discomforts of pregnancy and their management

These are all more marked in multiple pregnancy.

- Nausea and vomiting—more pronounced due to higher levels of β-HCG
  - Small frequent meals
  - Ginger preparations, pyridoxine, doxylamine
  - Oral antiemetics (e.g. metoclopromide, antihistamines, phenothiazines)
- Reflux oesophagitis
  - Avoid caffeine
  - Elevate bed head
  - Oral antacids—Mylanta
  - H_2 histamine receptor antagonists (e.g. cimetidine, ranitidine)

- Abdominal pressure and distension, discomfort
  - Rest (note routine bed rest for multiple pregnancies is not beneficial)
- Striae gravidarum
  - A vitamin E cream preparation may help
- Back pain
  - Rest, physiotherapy, water immersion
- Leg oedema and varicose veins
  - Compression stockings, elevation of lower limbs whenever possible

You supply Maria with information about the local multiple birth support group, which she is interested in contacting. Before she leaves your surgery, with a letter of referral to the hospital antenatal clinic, you also suggest to Maria that she and her husband might like to consider their options for family planning once this pregnancy is over. Natural family planning depends on a woman having regular cycles and being able to interpret the signs of ovulation. As Maria enters her 40s her periods may become less regular as progesterone levels decline. She may experience anovulatory cycles interspersed with normal cycles. Although she may wish to continue with the method, she should be aware of differences in how her body is functioning. Maria promises to discuss all this with her husband.

Clinical pearls

- Almost every minor and major side effect and complication of singleton pregnancy occurs with greater frequency in pregnancies with twins and higher multiples.
- Many women gain great psychological support and emotional benefit from contact with groups of other mothers who have experienced multiple births.

References and further reading

Hack KE, Derks JB, de Visser VL, et al. The natural course of monochorionic and dichorionic twin pregnancies: a historical cohort. Twin Res Hum Genet 2006; 9(3):450–5.

Society of Obstetricians and Gynecologists of Canada Practice Guidelines: Management of Twin Pregnancies parts 1 and 2: The Management of Nausea and Vomiting of Pregnancy; Guidelines for Prenatal Diagnosis. Available online at www.sogc.org.

Taylor MJ. The management of multiple pregnancy. Early Hum Dev 2006; 82(6):365–70.

White C. Fertility treatment regulator steps up warning about multiple births. BMJ 2006; 332(7554):1353.

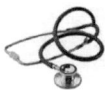

Case 13
Hazel and Kevin are trying for a pregnancy …

Hazel is a 38-year-old woman married for the first time 10 months ago. Her husband Kevin is aged 52. Kevin has been married previously and has two sons from that marriage but Hazel has never been pregnant and the couple have been trying to conceive since their marriage. Both partners come to consult you about the matter.

What are the important facts you wish to establish at the beginning of your history taking with this couple?

Hazel is now quite late in her reproductive years and if a problem with fertility exists she needs to be given help with this as soon as possible, whereas with younger women it is usual to wait for a full 12 months before commencing fertility investigations. It is important to establish that the couple are regularly achieving full sexual intercourse. Kevin is at an age at which erectile dysfunction is becoming increasingly common. Since his sons were conceived he may have experienced some health problem interfering with fertility or he may have undergone vasectomy and attempted reversal of this.

Initially you see both partners together. You then arrange to see and examine each partner individually. They are agreed that there is no problem achieving full intercourse and that this has occurred at least three to four times per week over the past 10 months. They are also agreed that they would wish to have some investigations if this seems appropriate but are not sure at this stage whether they would go as far as having in-vitro fertilisation (IVF). You explain to them that after the age of 40 Hazel statistically will quite rapidly become less likely to conceive and that even at age 38 she is less likely to do so spontaneously than when she was under 35. However, the chances of successful pregnancy are still quite high for the couple and IVF is certainly an increasingly successful possibility. You recommend that Hazel commence taking folic acid 0.5 mg daily.

At puberty there are about 250 000 potential ova in a woman's ovaries. In each cycle about 30 ova commence development but normally only one matures fully and is released in the process of ovulation; the remainder are spontaneously inhibited and absorbed. In the course of a woman's reproductive years she ovulates about 400 times—by the time she reaches her 40s most of these events of ovulation have been completed. Taking the oral contraceptive pill does not delay this process—degeneration of ova continues while a woman is on the pill.

What history do you take from Hazel?

You find that Hazel is in good general health. Her periods began at the age of 13 and for many years have been regular, 4–5 days in a 29-day cycle. She reports no dysmenorrhoea or dyspareunia. Her last period was 3 weeks previously. In her 20s she began taking the COCP and continued this with no problems until the age of 36; she has not been taking it recently. You confirm that Hazel has never been pregnant. She has no regular medications, no allergies, has had no serious illnesses or operations apart from a laparoscopic cholecystectomy at the age of 35, does not smoke cigarettes and drinks alcohol socially. She has never had a sexually transmitted infection. There is no relevant family history, in particular, no history of breast or ovarian cancer or of endometriosis. She last had a Pap smear, reported as normal, in your practice 2 years ago.

In taking a history from a woman presenting for investigation of fertility it is important to be sure that there have been no previous pregnancies, including ectopic pregnancies, pregnancies ending in miscarriage or induced abortion, and full-term pregnancies following which the baby was adopted. All of these have implications for current management. On occasion a woman may not wish to reveal previous pregnancy to her current partner; this desire must respected and the information kept confidential.

What examination do you perform for Hazel?

On examination Hazel appears healthy and neither over- nor underweight with her BMI in the healthy normal range; BP is 120/80 mmHg. There is no hirsutism, which might suggest PCOS, or galactorrhoea, which might suggest a raised prolactin level. You find nothing remarkable in the cardio-vascular or respiratory systems. You examine her abdomen—apart from the small scars of the cholecystectomy there is nothing of note detected.

Should you perform a vaginal examination for Hazel at this stage?

Yes—apart from giving useful information about the genital organs that may be relevant to her presenting problem, you will also be able to take the Pap smear, which is due.

You carry out a speculum examination looking at the vagina, which appears normal in colour and texture and 'well-oestrogenised'. The cervix also looks normal, with the central circular os characteristic of the nulligravida. You take a Pap smear. You then perform a bimanual pelvic examination. You find that the uterus feels somewhat enlarged with irregularities suggestive of fibroids, but there is no tenderness, either on palpating the uterus or on feeling in the lateral fornices, and no masses palpable in the fornices.

What history and examination do you undertake for Kevin?

Initially you will take a general medical history. You find that Kevin is also in reasonable health. He has been found to be hypertensive and to have elevated lipid levels; he currently takes a calcium channel blocker for hypertension and a statin to lower lipid levels. He has attended one of your partners recently for a check and both blood pressure and serum lipid levels have been found to be within the normal range. He admits to being overweight but a recent glucose tolerance test (GTT) has returned a normal result. He has two sons aged 24 and 20 by his first wife. Apart from an appendicectomy and an arthroscopy there is nothing else remarkable in his medical history. In particular, he has had no sexually transmitted infections, no testicular disease or surgery and has not had mumps.

> Type 2 diabetes is common in men in this age group, especially when obesity is present, and may be related both to erectile dysfunction and to subfertility. It is important to screen for diabetes in a presentation of this type if this has not recently been done.

Should you examine Kevin?

Yes—infertility involves two people. You should perform a general physical examination and a genital examination. However, it must be said that in practice it is quite common to arrange a semen analysis for the male partner and only proceed to examination if the results are abnormal.

On examination Kevin is normotensive and moderately overweight. There is no evidence of gynaecomastia. Secondary sex characteristics (i.e. facial hair, male pattern body hair distribution) are normal. Genital examination reveals normal-sized testes and penis. A vas deferens can be palpated bilaterally. There is a small, left-sided varicocele.

What investigations would you perform for Hazel and Kevin?

You organise some basic tests for Hazel and Kevin. Hazel needs an FBC and measurement of rubella and varicella antibody levels as part of

Investigations of female infertility/subfertility in general practice

Follicle stimulating hormone (FSH), luteinising hormone (LH)

- If these are elevated, this may indicate menopause or resistant ovary syndrome.
- If these are low, this may indicate pituitary hypogonadism (e.g. anorexia nervosa).

Prolactin

- Elevated serum prolactin interferes with pituitary function and may be due to a pituitary adenoma.

Serum androgens, sex hormone binding globulin

- Rarely, testosterone-secreting tumours of the ovary or adrenal gland can present as infertility. There are rare, and will more likely present as virilism.
- Polycystic ovarian syndrome (PCOS) is the most common cause of anovulatory infertility in women.

Thyroid function tests

- Both hyper- and hypothyroidism can cause anovulation.

pre-pregnancy screening, and a day 21 serum progesterone level test to see if this is in the ovulatory range. This result returns at 59 nmol/L, which is in the ovulatory range, so no further tests are required. If Hazel had not been ovulating, further tests would have been performed to delineate a cause. Note that these tests are often ordered routinely but are superfluous if ovulation has been proven. However, a pelvic ultrasound scan will give useful information about the size and shape of the uterus and ovaries.

Kevin requires a semen analysis. You explain to Kevin that this is best performed at a specialist andrology laboratory, which will provide a room for the collection. Alternatively, the specimen can be produced at home but must be delivered to the testing laboratory for examination within 2 hours. The specimen is produced by masturbation. You explain to Kevin that he must not have sexual intercourse or masturbate for at least 2 days prior to the test. As spermatogenesis takes approximately 3 months, an abnormal semen analysis may be a consequence of an illness during this time. Consequently, all abnormal semen analyses require repetition at 3 months.

Clinical comment

Semen analysis

Different laboratories may differ in their criteria but the following provides a guide:

- volume should be greater than 2.5 mL
- sperm count (actually sperm concentration) should be greater than 20 million per mL
- motility—more than 50% spermatozoa should be actively motile
- morphology—no more than 15% spermatazoa should be abnormal in microscopic appearance.

Finally, you explain to the couple that you may need to refer them to an infertility specialist gynaecologist for further assessment and possible infertility treatment. You explain that the specialist may want to assess whether Hazel's fallopian tubes are patent, and that this can be done in one of two ways. A hysterosalpingogram (HSG) is an X-ray performed while radio-opaque dye is injected into the uterine cavity via the cervix. If the fallopian tubes are patent, dye can clearly be seen outlining the tubal lumen and spilling from the tubes. Hysterosalpingogram using ultrasound is another method of assessing tubal patency. Alternatively, a laparoscopy can be performed to assess tubal patency, but this requires a general anaesthetic.

However, considering Hazel's age it is likely that the specialist will prefer to have ovarian volume assessed by USS to ascertain whether sufficient ova remain for an attempt at IVF, which is increasingly recommended for women experiencing difficulty with conception in their late 30s and early 40s, from any cause.

Clinical pearls

- Natural conception requires regular sexual intercourse with full vaginal penetration; the presence of healthy motile spermatozoa in the male; patent fallopian tubes and otherwise normal anatomy and regular ovulation in the female. Intercurrent health problems in either partner can interfere with conception. A good history and physical examination in general practice can identify many possible barriers to successful conception.

- It is important to emphasise to couples presenting with problems in conceiving that no procedure or treatment exists guaranteeing 100% success in achieving a pregnancy. Patients should be well informed about the details, risks and success rates of all investigations and procedures and given time to decide whether or not they wish to be referred for more invasive procedures. It is also worth noting that many infertility treatments are not fully reimbursed by Medicare.

References and further reading

Alesi R. Infertility and its treatment—an emotional roller coaster. Aust Fam Physician 2005; 34(3):135–8.

Bagshawe A, Taylor A. ABC of subfertility. Counselling. BMJ 2003; 327(7422):1038–40.

McLachlan RI, Yazdani A, Kovacs G, Howlett D. Management of the infertile couple. Aust Fam Physician 2005; 34(3):111–13, 115–17.

Quinn F. 'We're having trouble conceiving ...'. Aust Fam Physician 2005; 34(3):107–10.

Royal College of Obstetricians and Gynaecologists; National Evidence-Based Guidelines: Assessment and Treatment for People With Fertility Problems. Available online at www.rcog.org.uk.

Shaw RW, Souter WP, Stanton SL, eds. Gynaecology. 3rd edn. London: Churchill Livingstone, 2003:281–93.

Society of Obstetricians and Gynaecologists of Canada: Pregnancy Outcomes After Assisted Reproduction Technology. Available online at www.sogc.org.

Stewart J. Managing the subfertile couple. Practitioner 2004; 248(1663):742, 744–8.

Taylor A. ABC of subfertility: extent of the problem. BMJ 2003; 327(7412):434–6.

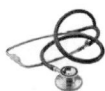

Case 14
Ruth complains of abdominal swelling …

Ruth is a 42-year-old woman who attends your practice intermittently. On this occasion she has come for a well-woman check and Pap smear. You note that the last time you saw her for such a check-up was more than 3 years ago. Ruth also tells you that she has been meaning to come for some time because she has been experiencing increasing lower abdominal discomfort, bloating and constipation, and is convinced that her abdomen is swollen—'my clothes don't fit any more'.

What are the important points in your history taking?

After taking details of the presenting complaint, a personal history of any cancer (breast, ovarian, bowel and endometrial in particular) should be asked about. Any change in menstrual cycles, any bowel symptoms, especially constipation and rectal bleeding, and any bladder symptoms, should also be inquired after. A family history of breast, bowel, endometrial and ovarian cancer should be noted.

Ruth reports unchanged regular cycles with no dysmenorrhoea and no dyspareunia. She is not experiencing any hot flushes or any mood changes but the lower abdominal symptoms mean she doesn't feel quite well. There is no known family history of breast or ovarian cancer. From your records you know that Ruth has two daughters, and that she underwent a laparoscopic sterilisation some 10 years ago. Ruth reports some constipation but states that this has been a recurrent problem for years. Apart from the bloating there is no other specific bowel complaint and no other relevant history.

What will be the most relevant parts of your physical examination?

You must look for signs of anaemia and lymphadenopathy, and carefully palpate the abdomen.

The conjunctivae and mucous membranes show no signs of anaemia and there are no palpable lymph nodes. Routine examination of the breasts reveals a firm very mobile lump about 1 cm diameter in the upper outer quadrant of the left breast.

Palpation of the abdomen shows a firm cystic swelling arising from the pelvis in the midline and tending towards the right lower quadrant. The swelling is non-tender and very mobile. The liver edge and the spleen are not palpable and there is no other abnormality detectable in the abdomen.

What is your tentative diagnosis?

An ovarian cyst is the most likely explanation here. A subserous fibroid on a narrow pedicle may produce the same findings. Other causes of a pelvic mass are less likely when the swelling is so mobile and feels cystic. To be absolutely certain that Ruth is not pregnant, you perform a urine β-HCG test—this is negative.

Causes of a pelvic mass

- Pregnant uterus—if in any doubt, perform a urine β-HCG test
- Fibroids or adenomyosis
- Ovarian tumour(s)—benign or malignant
- Pyosalpinx or hydrosalpinx or tubo–ovarian mass associated with PID
- Bladder—with chronic retention of urine
- Tumours arising from bladder or bowel

Will a vaginal examination be helpful in reaching a diagnosis?

Yes—you may be able to get a better idea of the size, consistency and anatomical relations of the mass. As well, Ruth is overdue for a Pap smear.

You perform a speculum examination for Ruth. The vagina appears normal and 'well-oestrogenised'; the cervix also appears healthy and you take a Pap smear. There is no abnormal discharge. You then perform a bimanual examination. This helps you decide that the mass is separate from the normally sized anteverted uterus, it is definitely cystic and can be balloted between your fingers, and appears to arise on the right side of the uterus. It partly balloons out of the right lateral wall of the vagina. The swelling is non-tender. It is about the size of a large grapefruit. These findings reinforce your clinical impression of a right ovarian cyst.

You explain these findings to Ruth and reassure her that everything you have felt points towards this being a benign cyst. You will arrange a pelvic ultrasound and some blood tests—FBC, urea and electrolyte levels and measurement of the tumour marker CA-125. You also arrange a mammogram and possible breast ultrasound.

It is important to look for tumour markers in any woman over the age of 30 presenting with a pelvic mass. The tumour marker most commonly associated with ovarian cancer is CA-125 (cancer antigen 125). However, remember that a negative result does not totally exclude ovarian cancer, nor does a positive result necessarily indicate malignancy—in particular, CA-125 may be elevated in endometriosis, pregnancy, pancreatitis and cirrhosis of the liver, as well as during menstruation. CASA (cancer-associated serum antigen), β-HCG, α-fetoprotein, LDH (lactate dehydrogenase) and inhibin are other tumour markers associated with ovarian cancers that may be helpful in diagnosis.

An FBC is an indicator of general health, and assessment of renal function is relevant to the presentation.

How do you arrange follow-up for Ruth?

Ruth returns to you in 2 days' time for the results of these tests. You have already made an appointment with a specialist gynaecologist, Dr Pepper, but have asked her to come back to discuss the results prior to that visit.

Ruth's blood test results are all within normal limits and the CA-125 level is well within the normal range. Her mammogram and subsequent breast ultrasound strongly suggest that the breast lump is a fibroadenoma. Arrangements are in place for her to attend the breast clinic the following day, when a fine-needle aspiration will be performed. Her pelvic ultrasound scan shows a normal-sized uterus and left ovary; the right ovary appears to have been completely replaced by a 9 cm cyst, which is loculated and in some places contains solid material. There is no free fluid in the pouch of Douglas. You reassure Ruth about these findings but explain that it will be necessary to remove the cyst surgically to make a definitive diagnosis and as treatment. The following week Ruth has a consultation with Dr Pepper and arrangements are made for laparotomy.

> A large ovarian cyst, especially one with solid components, is generally removed by laparotomy rather than laparoscopy to prevent intra-operational rupture of the cyst and the possible spill into the abdomen of malignant cells.

What is Ruth's subsequent progress?

You receive a discharge summary from Dr Pepper. At laparotomy through a Pfannenstiel incision the complete cyst and small amount of residual ovarian tissue has been removed. The capsule was smooth and unbroken. The left ovary was inspected and appeared normal, as did the uterus; these organs were conserved. Histological examination of the cyst has shown it to be a serous cystadenoma with no evidence of malignant change. Ruth has made an uneventful recovery.

Cytology of the breast biopsy obtained by fine-needle aspiration indicates that the lump is a fibroadenoma, and Ruth's Pap smear is reported as negative. Six weeks postoperatively you see Ruth again—she is well and symptoms have largely disappeared. You remind her of the importance of regular well-woman checks!

Clinical pearls

- Tumours of the ovary, including ovarian cancers, present late unless they are hormone-producing (rare) or undergo complications (e.g. haemorrhage, leaking or torsion of cysts). Bloating, swelling and vague abdominal discomfort is a common presentation; such symptoms should always be taken seriously.
- In considering the causes of a pelvic mass it is helpful to remember the five 'F's—fat, flatus, faeces, fetus and fluid.
- Women with a family history of ovarian and/or breast cancer should be offered genetic screening. Detection of the *BRCA* gene may lead to closer surveillance of the woman and of female relatives.

References and further reading

Gostout BA, Brewer MA. Guidelines for referral of the patient with an adnexal mass. Clin Obstet Gynecol 2006; 49(3):448–58.

Hogdall EV, Hogdall CK, Tingulstad S et al. Predictive values of serum tumour markers tetranectin, OVX1, CASA and CA125 in patients with a pelvic mass. Int J Cancer 2000; 89(6):519–23.

O'Connor V, Kovacs G, eds. Obstetrics, Gynaecology and Women's Health. Melbourne: Cambridge University Press, 2003:484–95.

Royal College of Obstetricians and Gynaecologists. Clinical Green-top Guidelines: Ovarian Cysts in Postmenopausal Women. Available online at www.rcog.org.uk.

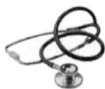

Case 15
Jamie-Lee needs to know about safe sex …

Jamie-Lee is a 16-year-old teenager who has been a patient of your practice since birth. Both her parents are also well known to you. Jamie-Lee is requesting contraceptive advice; in particular, she would like to start taking the COCP. She states that although she will tell her mother when she does start taking the 'pill', and does not believe her mother will object, she has not discussed this with her yet, and would feel embarrassed doing so.

How do you manage this consultation?

As well as addressing Jamie-Lee's specific request you should be assured about her general health. From previous records you know that Jamie-Lee has enjoyed good health, although she has asthma and uses salbutamol when required for this. On questioning she tells you that her periods began when she was 12, they are now regular and she does not have any dysmenorrhoea. Her last period finished a week ago. She also volunteers that she has been sexually active for the past 6 months.

What further history should be taken?

A full sexual history should be taken and Jamie-Lee made aware of the advantages and disadvantages of various forms of contraception. It is important also that you make sure that Jamie-Lee is aware of the need to practise safe sex, and how to do so—in particular, she should be aware of how and where to obtain condoms and how to use them. You should discuss cigarette smoking, and also ensure that no other health problems are overlooked, particularly any conditions that may be relative contraindications to prescribing the COCP.

Jamie-Lee tells you that she has had two sexual partners. She has been with her current boyfriend for 4 months and believes that the relationship is exclusive for both of them. She is aware of the need to use condoms except in relationships where both partners are monogamous. She tells you that with her first sexual partner she experienced reluctance to comply with condom use and on several occasions she had intercourse without protection. She smokes cigarettes at parties only, less than five per week—your strong advice to her is to quit altogether. There is nothing else she is aware of in her own medical history that might affect her suitability for the COCP.

What examination is required for Jamie-Lee?

Jamie-Lee is able to consent to examination herself although a chaperone should be present. Her blood pressure should be taken, a check of her heart and lungs and an abdominal examination performed. Since she has had unprotected sex she should have a vaginal examination and endocervical swabs taken; you explain the reasons for this to her.

> You advise Jamie-Lee that she should have a Pap smear carried out when she is about 18, and then every 2 years subsequently, in line with National Health and Medical Research Council (NHMRC) guidelines.

You carry out a full examination for Jamie-Lee, including vaginal examination, and note nothing remarkable. You take chlamydial swabs and swabs for gonorrhoea—both of these are taken from the endocervical canal just inside the external os. You prescribe a monophasic COCP, which Jamie-Lee can start immediately. You explain very clearly that she must not rely on this for contraceptive protection until she has taken seven active pills. You also emphasise the need for safe sex and the use of condoms unless both partners are exclusive in their sexual relationship.

> A first-catch urine specimen can be used for screening for chlamydia and gonorrhoea rather than endocervical swabs, although the test is not as sensitive as endocervical sampling.

Clinical comment

Precautions for women taking the COCP

- Remember to take the pill at the same time every day.
- If a pill is missed, take that pill as soon as it is remembered—barrier contraception will be needed for seven more active tablets.

- Gastrointestinal upsets may result in ineffective cover—barrier contraception and the 7-day rule apply.
- Broad-spectrum antibiotic use may also affect pill absorption and result in contraceptive failure—barrier methods should be used.
- A regular check of blood pressure should occur when obtaining a repeat prescription.
- Common and usual self-limiting side effects include breast tenderness, nausea and headaches.

What follow-up do you arrange for Jamie-Lee?

You ask Jamie-Lee to return in 3 months' time to see how she is progressing with the 'pill' and assure her that you are available to see her sooner if problems arise. You recommend that she tell her mother she is taking it but emphasise that your consultation with her is strictly confidential.

Three days later you receive the results of Jamie-Lee's swabs. The chlamydial screen (PCR) is positive. No other pathogens have been detected. Your receptionist is able to contact Jamie-Lee directly on her mobile phone and make another appointment. She presents looking extremely anxious and teary.

How do you manage this consultation?

You explain that chlamydia is a common infection. Certainly it is a sexually transmitted infection (STI) but it is treatable. In women chlamydia can be symptomless but it can cause infertility through salpingitis and subsequent tubal blockage. Chronic pelvic inflammatory disease (PID) that commences with a chlamydial infection is a common cause of chronic ill health in women.

> *'Who did I get it from?'* she wants to know

You reply that it is probably impossible to know the answer to this question at this stage, repeating that this is a common problem and really just requires correct management now. In principle she should contact all sexual partners and tell them of the diagnosis. She is upset at this and says that she could not face doing such a thing. She then admits to unprotected sex with her current partner. You strongly advise her telling him of her diagnosis and recommending that he seek attention from his own doctor. You prescribe

Summary of some common sexually transmitted infections—symptoms, signs, investigations and treatment in women

Infection	Symptoms	Signs	Investigations	Treatment
Gonorrhoea	Purulent vaginal discharge, urethral discharge, abdominal pain, pharyngitis, septic arthritis	Fever, Abdominal tenderness, Purulent cervical discharge	Swabs from endocervix, urethra, rectum, pharynx, First-catch urine for PCR	250 mg ceftriaxone IM in uncomplicated cases, full IV/oral antibiotic course for PID
Chlamydia	Often asymptomatic, Abdominal pain, vaginal discharge	Abdominal and pelvic tenderness, vaginal/cervical discharge	Swabs from endocervix, urethra, rectum, pharynx, First catch urine for PCR	Azithromycin 1 g in uncomplicated cases, prolonged doxycycline for PID
Herpes simplex (HSV 1 and2)	Skin tingling, blisters, painful ulceration, neuralgia, myopathy. Primary infection may be asymptomatic.	Fever, rashes, vesicles, blisters, ulceration	PCR or swab from lesion; viral culture	Aciclovir, valaciclovir, famciclovir for treatment and prophylaxis. Local treatment with lignocaine gel, ice packs, salt baths for relief of symptoms
Syphilis	Chancre, rashes, enlarged tender lymph nodes in early stages; latent phase symptomless; late disease cardiovascular neurological and psychiatric symptoms	Primary—chancre—hard painless genital nodule, Secondary—maculopapular rash, condylomata lata, Latent—symptomless (positive serology only)	RPR, VDRL tests for screening; *Treponema pallidum* haemagglutination antibody (TPHA), fluorescent treponemal antibodies (FTA-AbS) tests—*note*: once positive, always positive	Benzathine penicillin IM
Trichomoniasis	Often asymptomatic; may complain of discharge and/or odour	Frothy greenish-grey discharge with 'fishy' odour	Direct microscopic examination of wet preparation	Metronidazole or tinidazole
Human immunodeficiency virus (HIV)	Flu-like illness within two weeks of infection; malaise, fever, enlarged lymph nodes, Later weight loss, fever, malaise, fatigue, diarrhoea, enlarged nodes	Asymptomatic carrier state possible for many years, Fever, wasting, lymphadenopathy, specific infections (e.g. pneumonia) and malignancies (e.g. lymphoma)	HIV antibodies appear three month's after infection; once positive, always positive	Lifestyle management—diet, exercise, avoid smoking and recreational drugs, avoid or treat other STIs, Specific antiretroviral treatment, Treat intercurrent malignancy or pre-malignancy (e.g. cervical intra-epithelial neoplasia)
Genital warts	Warts in anogenital region, discharge, pain/discomfort, discharge	Visible warts on vulva, perineum, perianal area, cervix	Usually clinical examination only; biopsy if concern a lesion may be malignant	Local applications of podophyllin, 5-fluorouracil, imiquimod. Ablation using diathermy or cryotherapy, laser. Warts may disappear spontaneously

azithromycin for Jamie-Lee and arrange to see her again in 2 weeks' time for a further swab. You also recommend a fuller STI screen, including syphilis and HIV screening, which she agrees to.

Clinical pearls

- When one STI is diagnosed it is essential that a full STI screen, including screening for HIV, is offered together with contact tracing and appropriate counselling.
- Chlamydia infection is common among young sexually active women and has long-term implications for fertility and future health. Screening should be offered opportunistically when taking Pap smears and performing well-woman checks.

References and further reading

Freeto JP, Jay MS. 'What's really going on down there?' A practical approach to the adolescent who has gynecologic complaints. Pediatr Clin North Am 2006; 53(3):529–45, viii.

Miller KE. Diagnosis and treatment of Chlamydia trachomatis infection. Am Fam Physician 2006; 73(8):1411–16.

O'Connor V, Kovacs G, eds. Obstetrics, Gynaecology and Women's Health. Melbourne: Cambridge University Press, 2003:414–33.

Roberts TE, Robinson S, Barton P, et al. Screening for Chlamydia trachomatis: a systematic review of the economic evaluations and modelling. Sex Transm Infect 2006; 82(3):193–200.

Skidmore S, Horner P, Mallinson H. Testing specimens for Chlamydia trachomatis. Sex Transm Infect 2006; 82(4):272–5.

Society of Obstetricians and Gynaecologists of Canada. Sexual Health Counseling by Physicians. Available online at www.sogc.org.

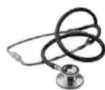

Case 16
Daniela has a molar pregnancy …

Daniela is a 25-year-old woman who has occasionally visited your practice. She has been trying to conceive for more than a year and has now succeeded. Her LMP is 10 weeks previously. She has irregular cycles and did not perform a home pregnancy test until 2 weeks previously—this was positive. However, she is now very anxious—this afternoon she noticed some slight vaginal bleeding, which has now increased in amount. She also reports almost constant nausea since the diagnosis of pregnancy was made.

What is your first step in the management of Daniela?

You take a history from Daniela. This is her first pregnancy. She has always had quite irregular menstrual cycles since her menarche at 12. Apart from her presenting complaints, she is well. In the past she has suffered from mild asthma using intermittent salbutamol, but has no other medical or surgical history, takes no other medication apart from folate and has no allergies. Daniela is of South-East Asian origin as is her partner Lee. Her mother is diabetic but there is no other relevant family history. Daniela has had a recent negative Pap smear.

What examination do you make for Daniela?

A general physical examination should be performed. Her BP is 110/70 mmHg, pulse rate is 70 bpm and she is afebrile. She does not exhibit any pallor. Heart sounds are normal. Examination of the abdomen shows some lower abdominal tenderness in the midline and a mass arising centrally from the pelvis, about the size of a 12-week pregnancy.

Do you perform a vaginal examination for Daniela?

Yes—you should visualise the cervix and perform a bimanual examination. Through the speculum you see a slightly open cervix with some dark blood trickling through the os. Bimanual examination confirms a 12-week size uterus with the os admitting a fingertip. The uterine size is therefore greater than you would expect for Daniela's pregnancy given the date of the LMP.

What possible explanations are there for this discrepancy?

It is possible that Daniela is wrong about the date of her last period, or that what she thought was a period was, in fact, bleeding associated with implantation of the pregnancy. It is also possible that she has a multiple pregnancy—on questioning she tells you that her mother's brothers are twins. Much less likely is gestational trophoblastic disease, either benign (a hydatidiform mole) or, very rarely, malignant (invasive mole or chorio-carcinoma).

How can you make a diagnosis here?

An ultrasound scan should be performed. You arrange this in the adjacent ultrasound practice requesting that it be performed urgently and you arrange to see Daniela again following the scan. Two hours later Daniela returns with the films—these show that no fetus is present and that there are numerous rounded echolucent areas seen: Daniela has a molar pregnancy.

How do you explain these findings to Daniela?

You explain to Daniela that she does not have a normal continuing pregnancy. She has an unusual condition but one more common in women of her ethnic background; in molar pregnancy the fetus has failed to develop but there is marked proliferation of the placental tissue. For further treatment you are going to refer Daniela for immediate consultation at your local hospital. You explain that molar pregnancy is completely treatable and that Daniela's prospects of having a subsequent normal pregnancy are high. You ensure that Daniela will be taken to the hospital by her partner, who will be there to support her.

> A woman having had a single molar pregnancy has a 1–1.5% risk of recurrence in subsequent pregnancies; a woman who has had two or more molar pregnancies has a 20% risk of recurrence in later pregnancies.

> *'What treatment am I likely to have at the hospital?'* Daniela
> wants to know

Further ultrasound scanning will be performed and quantitative β-HCG
levels will be measured as a baseline for treatment. The treatment of molar
pregnancy is evacuation of the contents of the uterus using suction curettage.
Subsequently, Daniela will need to have careful follow-up, with β-HCG levels
measured to ensure that these are dropping to normal levels and that there
is not persistent trophoblastic disease present.

Suction curettage of the uterus for molar pregnancy is best done
under ultrasound surveillance and with an intravenous infusion
of oxytocin running. Care must be taken to avoid perforating the
very soft vascular uterus that surrounds the pregnancy. Following
hydatidiform mole trophoblastic disease can persist—spread may
be local within the pelvis and/or there may be spread via the bloodstream to liver, lungs and brain. Hence, careful postoperative follow
up is indicated. For persisting or metastatic disease, cytotoxics, in
particular, methotrexate, have excellent response rates.

Six weeks later Daniela comes to see you again. You have received her
discharge letter from the hospital. After confirmation of the diagnosis by
USS and β-HCG levels, suction curettage has been performed. Histological
examination of the removed material has confirmed a complete hydatidiform
mole. Daniela has had weekly follow-up β-HCG levels performed by the
hospital; the last two have been negative. You are requested to continue
following Daniela with β-HCG levels monthly for 6 months and then
two-monthly for a further 6 months, communicating with the hospital. In
that time Daniela should avoid becoming pregnant as β-HCG levels from a
new pregnancy would make follow-up of the molar pregnancy impossible.
Daniela's name has been placed on the Central Mole Register of your state
to ensure and coordinate her follow-up.

Clinical comment

Hydatidiform mole may be complete or partial. With complete mole
no fetal parts are present; with partial mole fetal death usually occurs
followed by apparent miscarriage—often the diagnosis is made only with
histological examination of the products of conception.

Clinical pearls

- Molar pregnancy is uncommon but should not be forgotten when a woman presents with bleeding in early pregnancy or has a uterus which is 'large-for-dates'.
- Persistent trophoblastic disease is most common following a molar pregnancy but may occur after any pregnancy, including both early and late miscarriage and full-term delivery.

References and further reading

O'Connor V, Kovacs G, eds. Obstetrics, Gynaecology and Women's Health. Melbourne: Cambridge University Press, 2003:322–4.

Soper JT. Gestational trophoblastic disease. Obstet Gynecol 2006; 108(1):176–87.

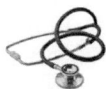

Case 17
Patricia complains of hot flushes …

Patricia is a 49-year-old legal secretary who comes to see you, concerned about hot flushes. These are worse at night, and she has difficulty sleeping and is tired and moody during the day. She tells you she is finding it hard to concentrate on her work—as she is responsible for managing a busy office this is causing her considerable anxiety.

What is the likely cause of her symptoms and what else do you need to ask?

Patricia is in the climacteric, approaching her menopause. Decreasing and fluctuating hormone levels are responsible for her symptoms. However, these may be exacerbated by other events or stresses in her life, or intercurrent medical conditions—none of these possible factors should be overlooked. You need to take a full history from Patricia.

Her presenting symptom, the flushes, have worsened over the past 2 months, waking her at night. She finds it difficult to get to sleep again, and begins to worry over problems that seem soluble in daylight hours. On further questioning you find that her father has recently died of a stroke. Her mother has had surgery for bowel cancer and is currently very dependent on her daughter. Patricia is the sole parent for two teenage boys, having been divorced for the past 5 years. Her older son is taking his final school examinations and is also learning to drive, two things that cause her concern. She admits to feeling depressed much of the time.

What further history do you take from Patricia?

You take a full menstrual history. Periods, she says, have become lighter over the past year but recently there have been episodes of bleeding between them; in fact, she's often not sure what's a period and what's not. She has kept a menstrual calendar over the past 2 months and when you examine this you see that Patricia has had bleeding for 2–3 days every week for the past 7 weeks. She also admits to some mild pelvic pain. Patricia has not been sexually active since her divorce. She has never had a sexually transmitted infection. From her notes you see that she last had a Pap smear in your practice 7 years previously, and she says she is sure she has not had one elsewhere in that time—'since the divorce I've tended to forget about sex and things like that', she tells you. She also tells you she has never had a mammogram.

In the past Patricia has had two full-term deliveries. She has had no significant illnesses. Apart from the removal of a thyroid cyst in her 20s, following which she did not require thyroxine therapy, she has had no surgery, takes no drugs apart from calcium and a multivitamin preparation, and is allergic to penicillin only. She does smoke 20 cigarettes a day and drinks three or four glasses of wine each night. On specific questioning she admits to drinking up to six cups of black coffee each day—'I need it to get through the day'. 'What about regular exercise?', you ask. She 'tries to get to the gym on Saturdays but doesn't always do so'.

What examination do you make for Patricia?

You carry out a general examination first. Patricia looks tired and drawn but otherwise well. She is slim, with a BMI of 24. Her blood pressure and examination of the heart and lungs are all within normal limits, inspection and palpation of the breasts is unremarkable and there is no lymphadenopathy. Abdominal examination reveals no abnormality.

You then proceed to a vaginal examination and pass a speculum in preparation for a Pap smear. To your surprise you see the strings of an IUCD protruding through the cervix. You tell Patricia of your finding and she is equally surprised. 'Good heavens', she says, 'I thought I had that out years ago, when my marriage was breaking up. Could that be the cause of the bleeding?' Indeed it could, you reply, and recommend removing the device, to which she agrees. You take the planned Pap smear prior to removing the IUCD so that bleeding does not contaminate the specimen. You also take swabs from the endocervical canal for microscopy and culture in case some mild infection is contributing to the bleeding. You then remove the IUCD without difficulty, identifying it as a copper-bearing IUCD, and you also take swabs from this.

Bimanual examination shows a slightly tender normal-sized uterus and you recommend to Patricia a course of oral antibiotics (metronidazole and cephalexin) as clinically she appears to have a degree of endometritis.

Intrauterine contraceptive devices

- IUCDs are safe, highly effective methods of contraception (Pearl Index 1 for copper-bearing IUCD, 0.1 for levonorgestrel-releasing IUCD).
- Copper-containing devices interfere with sperm motility, sperm and ovum transport, fertilisation and implantation; regular menstrual cycles continue and periods may be heavier than previously.
- Levonorgestrel-releasing devices thicken cervical mucus, decrease sperm motility and cause endometrial atrophy; oligomenorrhoea or amenorrhoea occurs in most women but may be preceded by several months of irregular spotting.
- PID is an uncommon complication of copper-bearing IUCDs, usually arising at the time of insertion; PID is rare with levonorgestrel-releasing IUCDs.
- Pain occurs in 1–2% of women, necessitating removal of the IUCD. Spontaneous expulsion occurs in 2–5% and may be unnoticed by the woman.
- It is important to remember that if pregnancy occurs in conjunction with the presence of an IUCD, it may be ectopic. If the pregnancy is intra-uterine there is a risk of septic miscarriage.

What is the next step in the care of Patricia?

You explain that normally with irregular bleeding around the time of the menopause you would refer her to a gynaecologist for full investigation. However, it seems likely that the retained IUCD was the cause of the bleeding, in which case removing it and giving antibiotics should improve the situation. You plan to send her for a transvaginal pelvic ultrasound scan to obtain a good view of the uterine cavity. You also order blood tests—FBC, FSH, thyroid function tests (TFTs) and liver function tests (LFTs)—and give her information about breast screening.

> FSH is the only hormone that needs measuring for the diagnosis of the climacteric. In many cases the diagnosis can be made on history alone.

What else should be discussed with Patricia?

You explain that you believe that the approach of the menopause is the main cause of Patricia's problems but that her lifestyle and family commitments are undoubtedly contributing to her anxiety and insomnia. You explain that short-term hormone therapy is a safe and sensible solution for her hot flushes but that until the cause of the irregular bleeding has been diagnosed prescribing this is contraindicated. You tell her that until her next consultation, which you schedule for a week's time, a mild hypnotic such as temazepam may be helpful. You would prescribe this only until she is established on hormone therapy and sleeping well again. You also suggest that she cut down on coffee, especially in the afternoons and evenings, and reduce her alcohol intake. She should also look at a suitable program for quitting cigarettes, which she should start once the immediate problems are solved. Regular exercise and diet also get a mention and you recommend that Patricia starts a calcium supplement of 1200 mg daily.

Patricia is happy with all this, says she is very relieved by what you have told her and agrees to return in a week. You supply her with written information about hormone replacement therapy.

How do you manage the second consultation?

At this consultation you immediately notice that Patricia looks brighter and less tired. She tells you that she is sleeping better but still has significant hot flushes during the day. You now have copies of all her results. The FBC and TFTs are within the normal range as are the LFTs, however, you take the opportunity to emphasise that her alcohol intake is above that considered safe for women. The FSH level is 60 mmol/L—well into the postmenopausal range. Ultrasound scan of the pelvis shows a thin endometrial strip 2 mm thick and no fibroids or polyps; the ovaries are small and show no abnormality. Swabs from the IUCD and cervical canal have shown a light growth of *Streptococcus faecalis*, which is sensitive to cephalosporins. Her Pap smear has been reported as normal.

You explain to Patricia that there is no obvious abnormality in the uterus and that almost certainly the cause of the bleeding was the continued presence of the IUCD. You can safely prescribe hormone replacement therapy, which she would like to try. She has no family history of breast cancer and has anyway made an appointment for a mammogram.

You commence her on a cyclical oral preparation of conjugated oestrogens and medroxyprogesterone acetate and arrange to review her in 2 months. You warn her that she may have some slight breakthrough bleeding on this for the first few months but that this should settle down and she should have light withdrawal bleeds subsequently. She may also experience some nausea or headache, which should be self-limiting. It will take up to 4 weeks for the hot flushes to subside completely; in this time she will stop the temazepam.

Patricia returns to see you in 2 months' time. She is now looking extremely well and happy. What are the important points in this consultation?

Patricia tells you that she has had only slight withdrawal bleeding since commencing the hormone therapy. The lower abdominal pain that she had been experiencing has also completely disappeared, as have her hot flushes. Her mammogram showed no abnormality. Work is now manageable, her son has passed his driving test and seems to be acting responsibly and her mother has gone on a cruise with a friend to Fiji. Life is looking good.

'How long can I stay on the hormones?' she asks

You explain that it is safe to continue with hormone therapy in the short term to deal with the period of time in which the hot flushes and other menopausal symptoms are most debilitating. She can be switched to continuous therapy if she wishes in view of the scanty withdrawal bleeds and her elevated FSH. In 12–18 months she can try weaning herself off the therapy, although if she finds her symptoms return she can continue for several years, under medical supervision. You explain that there has been shown to be slight increases in the risks of breast cancer and of thromboembolic incidents with long-term hormone therapy (greater than 5 years) and that studies have not shown any cardiac benefit from its use. It does, however, protect long-term against osteoporosis. Since publication of the largest study into long-term hormone replacement therapy, there has been a tendency not to prescribe it, but the pendulum has now swung back cautiously and it may be useful in some women in the long term. Meanwhile, she can continue with her preparation quite safely, returning for a further check-up in a year's time, and reporting back if she has any problems, particularly vaginal bleeding.

Patricia also tells you that she has taken up a Pilates class three times a week, and arranged to join a church group dedicated to quitting smoking.

Clinical pearls

- Hormonal therapy should be tailored to the particular requirements of the individual woman and may be modified as a woman passes from the perimenopausal to the postmenopausal period.
- Lifestyle factors may be important in exacerbating symptoms and should always be inquired about. Weight loss, attention to diet, regular exercise, stopping smoking, reducing alcohol and coffee intake, and taking measures to reduce stress may all improve a woman's sense of wellbeing at this time of life.

References and further reading

Heikkinen J, Vaheri R, Timonen U. A 10-year follow-up of postmenopausal women on long-term continuous combined hormone replacement therapy: update of safety and quality-of-life findings. J Br Menopause Soc 2006; 12(3):115–25.

O'Connor V, Kovacs G, eds. Obstetrics, Gynaecology and Women's Health. Melbourne: Cambridge University Press, 2003:519–27.

Prentice RL, Langer RD, Stefanick ML et al. Combined analysis of Women's Health Initiative observational and clinical trial data on postmenopausal hormone treatment and cardiovascular disease. Am J Epidemiol 2006; 163(7):589–99.

Shaw RW, Souter WP, Stanton SL, eds. Gynaecology. 3rd edn. London: Churchill Livingstone, 2003:415–28.

Travers C, O'Neill SM, Khoo SK, King R. Hormones down under: hormone therapy use after the Women's Health Initiative. Aust N Z J Obstet Gynaecol 2006; 46(4):330–5.

Wathen CN. Health information seeking in context: how women make decisions regarding hormone replacement therapy. J Health Commun 2006; 11(5):477–93.

Women's Health Intitative 2002. Risks and benefits of estrogen plus progestin in healthy postmenopausal women. JAMA 2002; 288:321–33.

Case 18
Debbie presents with some irregular bleeding …

Debbie is a woman of 48 who is referred to you by the women's health nurse who conducts well-women checks in small towns in your region. Debbie has not had a Pap smear for 12 years. She was divorced when she was 40 and has been sexually active only infrequently since that time. She believed that she did not need Pap smears if she was not having regular sex. She presented to the women's health nurse because she had some bloodstained discharge. The nurse was concerned by the appearance of Debbie's cervix on speculum examination.

What is your first step in the management of this case?

Take a full history. Debbie tells you that her periods seemed to have stopped when she was 47. She had some hot flushes at that time, which soon settled. Then she began to have slight irregular bleeding, which she decided was part of 'the change'. More recently she has had a bloodstained discharge that has been offensive at times and she felt that this was not normal. There has been no pain associated with the bleeding or discharge.

What further information do you need from Debbie?

Debbie informs you that she has had five children with three different partners—all normal pregnancies and deliveries. She has been married and divorced twice. She lives on her own, all her children having left home. She works as a waitress in a country pub and lives on the job. She smokes 30 cigarettes a day and drinks socially. She had her appendix removed at the age of 14. In the past 10 years she has had a cholecystectomy and a hospital admission for low back pain—she states that on neither occasion was a Pap smear suggested. She takes occasional analgesics for backache but no other regular medications and has no allergies. Her mother died from breast cancer at age 60 and she has had several mammograms since the age of 40 as she has been concerned about getting breast cancer herself.

You take the opportunity to counsel Debbie about the effects of cigarette smoking on her health and offer her help with giving up cigarettes.

Cervical cancer is associated with early age at first intercourse, number of sexual partners, cigarette smoking and use of the COCP; however, it is also known that high-risk HPV types are necessary, although not sufficient, for the development of HSIL and cervical cancer.

What examination do you perform for Debbie?

General examination is performed first. Debbie is a rather underweight woman who looks generally well but there is some clubbing of the fingers of both hands and some moist sounds on auscultation of her chest. Her BP is 120/85 mmHg, pulse is 68 bpm and she is afebrile. There is no lymphadenopathy in the cervical, supraclavicular or inguinal nodes.

Examination of the abdomen shows the scars expected from her surgery. There is no hepatomegaly or splenomegaly. There are no intra-abdominal masses and no tenderness.

What is your next step?

You perform a vaginal examination. Speculum examination shows a fungating growth about 3 cm in diameter on the anterior lip of the cervix. This bleeds on touch with the brush you use to take a Pap smear. The lesion on bimanual palpation is firm and nodular and anteriorly reaches forward towards the vaginal wall. The uterus itself is mobile and anteverted.

It is important whenever a Pap smear is taken that the cervix is completely and carefully inspected. Pap smears may fail to make the diagnosis in the presence of frank cervical cancer because much of the surface epithelium around the cancer is necrotic.

Debbie is now very worried, and asks you if she has cancer. What do you tell her?

It is important to tell Debbie the truth in as detailed a way as you think appropriate. You explain that the women's health nurse has correctly noticed an unusual growth on the cervix. You feel that, yes, this is possibly an early cervical cancer. You will be referring Debbie promptly to a gynaecologist in the nearest large town who will take over investigations and subsequent management if the diagnosis is confirmed. You will also help Debbie make whatever social and work arrangements are needed while she undergoes investigation and treatment.

'What kind of investigations?' Debbie asks

There will be an initial history and examination as already performed by you. The next steps will include blood tests (FBC, urea and electrolytes, liver function tests [LFTs]), ultrasound scan of her pelvis and kidneys, chest X-ray, examination under anaesthesia (EUA) and biopsy of the cervical lesion, cystoscopy, and possibly computed tomography (CT) or magnetic resonance imaging (MRI). All of these, you explain, will be to determine whether the cancer has spread. Debbie can then expect to have the results of all these tests explained to her in detail and treatment offered.

Clinical comment

Cervical cancer

In more than 95% of cases cervical cancer is of squamous origin; adeno-carcinoma of the cervix is, however, becoming more common. Cervical cancer spreads directly to the vagina, bladder and rectum (rarely to the ovary); by the lymphatics (iliac nodes then para-aortic nodes); and by the bloodstream (to liver, lungs, bones). Cystoscopy provides information about bladder involvement. MRI is increasingly being used to measure tumour volume and size; CT scanning is used for the assessment of pelvic lymph nodes. Once the primary tumour reaches 4 cm in size there is a 40% chance of lymph node involvement and this is the reason for the relatively poor survival figures for this cancer.

'Will I need an operation?' Debbie asks

It is likely that Debbie will be recommended a radical hysterectomy with resection of the pelvic lymph nodes. If investigations show that the primary tumour is larger than 4 cm diameter, then a combination of radiotherapy and chemotherapy will be more appropriate. Recent views of treatment are to offer either surgery or chemoradiation to reduce the severity of side effects concomitant on multiple therapies.

Results for the treatment of cervical cancer range from 95–100% for 5-year survival in patients with stage I cancer to only 10% 5-year survival for women with involvement of the bladder and/or rectal mucosa at the time of the first diagnosis.

Clinical pearls

- All women receiving medical care for any condition whatsoever should be offered Pap smears opportunistically or, if this is not feasible, reminded of the importance of regular smears. Cervical cancer is one of the few cancers that, if detected in its premalignant or early stages, has close to 100% cure rates.
- All women who smoke cigarettes should receive advice about the effects of smoking on health, and offered help with quitting, on every occasion on which they present to health-care providers.
- All women with irregular vaginal bleeding, whether pre-, peri- or postmenopausal, should have prompt examination and investigation to outrule malignancy.

References and further reading

Kesic V. Management of cervical cancer. Eur J Surg Oncol 2006; 32(8):832–7.

Ngoma T. World Health Organization cancer priorities in developing countries. Ann Oncol 2006; 17 (suppl. 8):viii9–viii14.

Selman TJ, Prakash T, Khan KS. Quality of health information for cervical cancer treatment on the internet. BMC Womens Health 2006; 20(6):9.

Shaw RW, Souter WP, Stanton SL, eds. Gynaecology. 3rd edn. London: Churchill Livingstone, 2003:583–95.

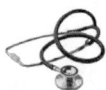

Case 19
Miranda fears she may be pregnant …

Miranda is a 19-year-old student who is a long-time patient of your practice. Her family is also well known to you. Miranda arrives the moment the practice doors open at 8 am on the Tuesday following a long weekend and asks for an urgent appointment. She appears anxious and distressed to your reception staff so, despite a heavy schedule, you agree to squeeze her in—your first booked patient has not arrived. You take a quick look at Miranda's notes and see that one of your partners last saw her 6 months previously for a well-woman check and a prescription for the COCP. Her Pap smear taken then was negative. Otherwise, apart from common childhood illnesses, Miranda has been in good health.

Miranda sits down in your consulting room and bursts into tears

'I've been really stupid', she says. 'I went away for the weekend with some friends, not expecting to have sex, but that's what happened. I stopped the pill two months ago because I broke up with Chris so I didn't use anything. Now I've got this discharge and burning, I'm afraid I've got something awful and I could be pregnant.'

How do you deal with this situation?

You explain calmly that these are common situations and there are solutions that can be offered. Firstly, you need to take a history from Miranda.

Her LMP was 3 weeks previously. She has had three periods since discontinuing the COCP, including the withdrawal bleed immediately following the last active tablet. Her cycle seems to be re-establishing with 4 days of bleeding every 27 days.

Miranda has had unprotected intercourse with a new partner on the Saturday evening, Sunday and Monday mornings of the previous weekend.

The first episode was about 10 pm on Saturday, that is, about 58 hours prior to your consultation. She assures you that she has not been otherwise sexually active for more than 2 months.

Since Sunday evening she has been experiencing vaginal burning and now has a white vaginal discharge.

What other history do you take from Miranda?

Miranda has never had a sexually transmitted infection previously and she has never been pregnant. She takes no medications, has no allergies and has no other relevant medical history.

What do you now tell Miranda?

You explain to Miranda that emergency contraception is readily available to her—in fact, it can be obtained over-the-counter from pharmacists without a prescription. You would recommend a regimen of two tablets of levonorgestrel each of 750 µg. The first should be taken as soon as possible—you suggest that she goes immediately after the consultation to the adjacent pharmacy to obtain the tablets. The second should be taken 12 hours later—at 9 pm that evening.

'Is it 100% effective?' she asks. *'And are there any side effects?'*

If taken within 72 hours of unprotected intercourse, you tell Miranda, the levonorgestrel regimen is 75–85% effective at preventing pregnancy. Put another way, 2% of women having unprotected intercourse and taking the tablets will still become pregnant. You also point out that from her history Miranda would have been on day 19 of her cycle, about 6 days post-ovulation in what is probably another 27-day cycle, at the time of first intercourse, so that her chances of pregnancy are thereby reduced.

> Emergency contraception will not dislodge or abort an established, implanted pregnancy. Levonorgestrel is not teratogenic—if a pregnancy has occurred from an earlier act of unprotected intercourse, there is no risk to the fetus.

Other forms of emergency contraception

Yuzpe method

- Two tablets containing ethinyloestradiol 50 µg and levonorgestrel 250 µg are given within 72 hours of unprotected intercourse and repeated in 12 hours. Tablets containing these doses of oestrogen and progestogen are no longer available in Australia so, alternatively, four tablets each containing 30 µg ethinyloestradiol and 150 µg levonorgestrel may be used, again repeated in 12 hours. Nausea and vomiting due to the high dose of oestrogen may result from this regimen and an anti-emetic may be needed. There is a failure rate of 2–3% with this method.
- Mifepristone 10 mg can be given within 5 days of unprotected intercourse and is as effective as the progesterone-only method; however, it is not yet available in Australia.

Insertion of a copper-bearing IUCD within 5 days of unprotected intercourse will be effective at preventing pregnancy, with a failure rate of 1%. There is the advantage of a continuing contraceptive effect; however, it is not the contraceptive method of choice in a young nulliparous woman, particularly when there is the possibility of a concurrent STI.

What further advice do you give Miranda with regard to the possibility of pregnancy?

You tell Miranda that her period may occur earlier than expected and that the subsequent cycle may be longer than normal. If she does not get her period by the expected date she should have a pregnancy test, which she can do herself with an over-the-counter kit or by returning to your surgery. You point out that she is unlikely to be pregnant but that if she has a positive pregnancy test she should return as soon as possible to discuss her options.

You must also discuss future contraception. She tells you that the encounters of the weekend may develop into an ongoing relationship. She has a supply of the COCP at home but would also like information about other hormonal forms of contraception.

You explain to her the details of the two forms of progestogen-only contraception, apart from the mini-pill, currently available in Australia and suitable for Miranda: medroxyprogesterone acetate injections and the etonogestrel implant. You mention the levonorgestrel-releasing IUCD but explain that it is more suited to women having had one or more children.

> You must also consider Miranda's second concern, the vaginal discharge, and her fear that she may have contracted a sexually transmitted infection. How do you deal with this question?

You should conduct an examination for Miranda and offer a full STI screen. You find Miranda to be generally well and abdominal examination shows no abnormality. You proceed to vaginal examination and pass a speculum. There is a curdy white discharge suggesting *Candida* infection. Otherwise, the vagina and cervix appear unremarkable. You take swabs from the upper vagina—a high vaginal swab for *Candida* and trichomoniasis—and also from the endocervical region for chlamydia and gonorrhoea. (Wet preparations on slides for direct examination can also be used if facilities are available for the immediate diagnosis of candidiasis and trichomoniasis, however, they have low sensitivity at detecting these conditions.)

You also arrange for Miranda to have initial serological screening for syphilis, HIV and hepatitis B. Follow-up serology should also be arranged. You give Miranda a further appointment in 7 days' time for the results of these tests but suggest that meanwhile she buy an over-the-counter preparation for 'thrush' (candidiasis) as you feel that this is the most likely cause of her symptoms. A single-dose regimen is likely to be highly effective.

What other advice do you give Miranda?

You take the opportunity to remind Miranda of the importance of safe sex. Using condoms, you tell her gently, not only greatly reduces the chances of pregnancy, it also can prevent or reduce the chances of transmission of STIs.

Condoms—use and effectiveness

- A condom should be applied before any sexual penetration occurs.
- Only water-based lubricants should be used with condoms.
- Following ejaculation and withdrawal, the condom should be removed by holding the rolled rim and drawing it carefully from the erect penis before detumescence occurs.
- Condoms can deteriorate and may be ineffective if brittle or sticky. Condoms should never be reused.
- Condoms are highly effective if used properly and consistently— Pearl Index 3. Effectiveness is increased if they are used with spermicides.
- The female condom, if used correctly, is equally effective and also protects more fully against STIs.
- Both male and female condoms should be disposed of safely.

Clinical pearls

- Information about condom use should be supplied opportunistically in all consultations dealing with contraception and STIs.
- Condoms provide effective contraception and effective protection against STIs if used appropriately and consistently.

References and further reading

Abbott J, Feldhaus KM, Houry D et al. Emergency contraception: what do our patients know? Ann Emerg Med 2004; 43(3):376–81.

Goulard H, Moreau C, Gilbert F. Contraceptive failures and determinants of emergency contraception use. Contraception 2006; 74(3):208–13.

Hamoda H, Ashok PW, Stalder C et al. A randomized trial of mifepristone (10 mg) and levonorgestrel for emergency contraception. Obstet Gynecol 2004; 104(6):1307–13.

Merchant RC, Damergis JA, Gee EM et al. Contraceptive usage, knowledge and correlates of usage among female emergency department patients. Contraception 2006; 74(3):201.

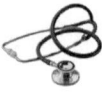

Case 20
Sunithra is depressed following the birth of her baby …

Sunithra is a 36-year-old patient of your practice who gave birth to her first baby 6 weeks previously at your local hospital. She has been a patient of your practice since she was a teenager, so you know her very well. She had been trying to conceive for several years, and this pregnancy was the result of several IVF attempts. Sunithra was delighted to be pregnant, but was very anxious during the pregnancy. You provided her antenatal care, sharing this with the hospital. You have received a discharge summary from the hospital stating that Sunithra gave birth to a healthy baby girl by emergency caesarean section, birth weight 3570 g. Sunithra is seeing you today for her 6-week routine postnatal check. You have been somewhat surprised that she has not come by to show you and your staff her new baby, as she promised to do so before the birth. On checking her medical records, you see that she is due for her next routine Pap smear.

The first consultation

Sunithra enters the room without her baby, looking very tired and flat. She doesn't give you the normal bright greeting you've come to expect from her over the years. You ask her how she is, and has she brought her baby, as you'd really been looking forward to seeing her.

'I'm OK, doctor. I've left Kamala at home because she is having another one of her crying fits, and I didn't want to bring her today.' Sunithra flops into her chair and looks exhausted. You ask her if she is getting enough rest. 'Not really. I was exhausted after the birth and she cries a lot. I haven't really been getting much sleep.' Her husband has been trying to help but because she has been off work he is working extra shifts at the factory to help their finances. Her mother has come from interstate for the birth, but Sunithra's relationship with her mother has always been difficult and she feels her mother's presence is not of much benefit. 'She's critical of everything, and everything is always my fault—the baby crying, the breastfeeding problems, the caesarean—she makes me feel like a total failure.' At this point Sunithra starts crying uncontrollably.

What are your concerns in this situation and how do you proceed?

You offer her some tissues and a comforting hand, and when she stops crying ask further about her problems. You make it clear that this will be a prolonged consultation and you have plenty of time to listen. Sunithra tells you that her husband hasn't really been at home much, and she finds it hard to confide in him, particularly with her mother being present. She had to have an emergency caesarean section for obstructed labour, and she feels as if she has somehow failed as a woman. Breastfeeding is proving to be very difficult, and she does not know who to turn to for help.

You decide that you will defer the Pap smear until a later visit, as Sunithra's other concerns are more pressing. However, you do examine her abdomen and confirm the caesarean section incision is well healed, with no evidence of infection. You perform a breast examination—Sunithra's nipples are both cracked and inflamed.

What immediate practical help can you offer to Sunithra?

You explain to Sunithra that she needs some more help and support, and arrange this by referring her to the local day centre for new mothers, where a lactation consultant visits to provide assistance with breastfeeding. You advise her that she should probably thank her mother for her help, but suggest that she is no longer required and should return home. You explain to Sunithra that both she and the baby are healthy, and that she should not feel as if she has failed by requiring a caesarean section. It is most important that she not blame herself for this outcome. You go over the indications for the caesarean with her—the operation was performed for a good medical reason: she was not progressing in labour. You explain that this is a common scenario with a first labour, not something that is anyone's fault, and that modern surgery is available expressly to deal with such problems.

You then arrange to see Sunithra in 1 week's time to see how she is getting along, and ask her to bring Kamala too so you can perform her 6-week baby check.

Breastfeeding problems are common. Most hospitals have lactation consultants—midwives who specialise in breastfeeding and its difficulties and are freely available to help and encourage new mothers. As well, many cities have mother and baby day centres to help postnatal women with these common difficulties.

The second consultation

One week later Sunithra returns to see you. Again, she has not brought Kamala. Your receptionist tells you that the baby has been left at home with Sunithra's husband, because 'she was crying too much'. You have heard from the day centre that despite their best efforts Sunithra has stopped trying to breastfeed. At this visit Sunithra appears remote and withdrawn, and answers your questions in a monosyllabic fashion. She is somewhat unkempt with unwashed hair and crumpled clothing, which concerns you as she is usually fastidious about her appearance. As she is not volunteering anything spontaneously, you start asking her specific questions:

'How is Kamala?'—no reply.
'Has you mother gone home?'—she grunts, 'Yes, thank goodness.'
'How is your husband?'—no reply.
'Have you been sleeping well?'—'No, it's hard to get to sleep and I wake up early and can't get back to sleep.'
'How is your appetite?'—'I have no appetite.'
'Have you been having any bad or negative thoughts?'—'Like what?'
'How do you feel about Kamala?'—'I don't feel anything about her. I hate it when she cries. I don't feel any love or maternal instincts. I hate it when she cries—it must mean I'm a bad mother if I don't feel anything for her. Sometimes I feel as if I want to hurt her to make her quiet!'
'How do you feel about yourself? Have you had any thoughts of hurting yourself?'—'Sometimes I just want to die—I feel like a bad mother. No normal mother would feel these things.'
'Have you tried hurting yourself or the baby?'—'No.'
'Have you told anyone about these feelings?'—'No.'
'Are you hearing any voices telling you bad things?'—'No.'

What are your conclusions and concerns from this interview?

Clearly, Sunithra has significant postnatal depression. You are very concerned about her welfare, and that of Kamala. You decide to call her husband Ranjit and ask him to come up to the surgery. He brings Kamala, who does indeed cry lustily for the entire time they are both there. You explain to both Sunithra and Ranjit that she has severe postnatal depression, and that you are worried about her. Sunithra bursts into tears and becomes incoherent. In part, she does seem relieved that this is all out in the open. However, you are very concerned that she and Kamala need supervised care and that she herself needs specialist psychiatric treatment.

> Postpartum depression is common, affecting about 13% of women; the peak period of onset is 4–6 weeks postpartum but it can occur at any time in the first year of the infant's life. About 80% of women will experience mood lability and anxiety (the 'baby blues') on days 3–4 postpartum; this is best managed by sympathetic support and anticipation of the condition in antenatal classes, and is self-limiting. Postpartum psychosis is rare, affecting 1–3 women per thousand.

What practical measures do you take?

You ring your local hospital, which has a mother and baby unit within their psychiatry department. You arrange for Sunithra and Kamala to be admitted immediately. Sunithra is assessed by the consulting psychiatrist and commenced on selective serotonin reuptake inhibitor (SSRI) antidepressants. She remains in the unit for 3 weeks. At the end of that time you receive a call from the nursing staff to ask that you follow her up in the next few days. You ring Ranjit to arrange an appointment to see the entire family in 2 days time.

> Many cities have special mother and baby units within psychiatric departments. These are ideal for the treatment and observation of mothers and babies, although waiting lists may be long. In smaller centres such services may not exist, but it is important to ensure that the mother and baby remain together if possible, and that they are both safely supervised.

> Antidepressants make take 2–3 weeks to be effective, and mood may deteriorate within that interval. It is in this time that self-harm or harm to the baby is a strong possibility. Antidepressant medications have been used in lactating women but ethical considerations limit the implementation of randomised controlled trials; specialist advice should be sought in this situation.

The third consultation

Two days later you meet the entire family, and Sunithra looks more like her old self. Her mood seems much better, and she is able to smile once or twice. She clearly adores Kamala, who seems much calmer too, and cuddles her throughout the consultation.

She now says, 'Thank you for looking after me, doctor. I felt so alone and frightened. I couldn't talk about this to anyone because I didn't want them to think I was mad, or evil. I was so scared about hurting Kamala.'

Is Sunithra now at risk of harming herself or her baby?

You can see that this is now not a likely scenario, which is also the psychiatrist's opinion. You institute the follow-up plan suggested by the psychiatrist, and make sure Sunithra knows she has someone to call if she is concerned. You reiterate this point to Ranjit as well. Relieved that all appears well, you make arrangements with Sunithra to perform her long-delayed '6-week visit' baby check and Pap smear.

Clinical pearls

- Postpartum depression is common, affecting about 13% of women, and may have profound and long-lasting effects on the woman, her child and her family as a whole. Early detection and ongoing supervision are essential to achieve the best possible outcome for all involved.
- Sometimes women feel as if they have 'failed' if they have not had a perfectly normal uncomplicated birth. About 30% of women having a first baby will have a caesarean section or instrumental vaginal birth. It is important to emphasise that a healthy mother and baby are the desired outcome, and that this cannot and does not have to

be achieved through a spontaneous vaginal birth for every woman. Feelings of worthlessness and failure are common and should be actively addressed. It is most important to explain the reasons behind the decisions which led to the intervention, and reassure the woman that she must not blame herself, and has not failed at motherhood if a vaginal birth did not eventuate. Sometimes, a debriefing session with the hospital or obstetrician who was involved may be worth considering.

References and further reading

Beck CT. Postpartum depression: it isn't just the blues. Am J Nurs 2006; 106(5):40–50.

Blenning CE, Paladine H. An approach to the postpartum office visit. Am Fam Physician 2005; 72(12):2491–6.

Creasy R, Resnik R, eds. Maternal–Fetal Medicine—Principles and Practice. 5th edn. Philadelphia: WB Saunders, 2004:1193–8.

Gavin NI, Gaynes BN, Lohr KN et al. Perinatal depression: a systematic review of prevalence and incidence. Obstet Gynecol 2005; 106(5 Pt 1):1071–83.

Howard L. Postnatal depression. Clin Evid 2005; (14):1764 75.

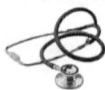

Case 21
Sara would like to be pregnant …

Sara is a 28-year-old woman who comes to see you for a well-woman check but also has a number of other issues to discuss.

Sara is already well known to you, having been a patient of your practice for at least 10 years. From the age of 18 she took the COCP, both for contraception and for the control of heavy painful periods. At 24, having been married a year, she stopped the 'pill' with the intention of trying to become pregnant. However, within 9 months her periods were again very heavy and irregular, she had not conceived and was, in fact, experiencing some deep dyspareunia that was making her attempts to conceive difficult. You referred her to a gynaecologist, Dr Pepper, who performed a laparoscopy and found a moderate degree of endometriosis. Areas of endometriosis particularly on the uterosacral ligaments were resected and subsequently Sara elected to have a 6-month course of medroxyprogesterone. 'I was fed up with bleeding all the time,' she said. 'I wanted some time to think over the whole thing.' Two years ago at the time of her last well-woman check she decided to go back on the COCP for at least a year before trying again to conceive. You renewed her prescription last year when she was well and have not seen her since.

Endometriosis may be asymptomatic but when symptoms occur they are characteristically pelvic pain, dysmenorrhoea, deep dyspareunia, menorrhagia and infertility. Small areas of endometriosis may cause severe symptoms (e.g. nodules of endometriosis on the uterosacral ligaments may be the cause of severe dyspareunia); conversely, large areas of endometriosis with extensive pelvic adhesions may be asymptomatic. A definite diagnosis of endometriosis can only be made at laparoscopy or laparotomy, although the condition may be suspected from the history; there is also a familial tendency to endometriosis.

At this consultation Sara tells you that she stopped the COCP 4 months ago. 'My periods are back,' she says, 'regular but not heavy and quite manageable. However, I'm still not pregnant although we're trying, and I'm afraid I've got this discharge …'

What history do you take from Sara?

She tells you that the discharge is watery and occasionally pink, not offensive and not burning, stinging or itching. It is most profuse after sex, and she finds this embarrassing and uncomfortable. She is absolutely certain there is no possibility of a sexually transmitted infection, and denies that either she or her partner has ever had an STI. She has been well since her last consultation with you; apart from her endometriosis and its associated symptoms Sara has always enjoyed good health. She is on no medications, has had no surgery apart from the laparoscopy, does not smoke and has no allergies. Since she has been trying to conceive she has abstained from alcohol and takes folic acid daily. Her partner, who is a patient of your practice, is also in good health, although he has never had semen analysis performed.

What examination do you make for Sara?

You perform a short general examination, including blood pressure and auscultation of the heart. You inspect and palpate the abdomen, finding nothing remarkable, in particular, no lower abdominal tenderness or masses. You then perform a vaginal examination.

What are your expected findings on vaginal examination?

Given that a discharge related to an STI is unlikely, there is the possibility of *Candida* infection or a cervical ectopy associated with COCP use. In addition, occasionally specks of endometriosis are seen on the cervix.

On passing a speculum, however, what you observe is a large cervical polyp protruding on a stalk through the cervical os. This is very mobile but it is not possible to see the top of the stalk. On moving the polyp aside to take the Pap smear you also note a moderate degree of cervical ectopy (ectropion) as expected in a woman who has been taking the COCP. The polyp appears benign.

Causes of vaginal discharge

- Physiological discharge—may be more marked when a degree of cervical ectropion (ectopy) is present
- Infections—cervical (chlamydia, gonococcal) or vaginal (*Candida*, trichomoniasis, bacterial vaginosis, group B streptococci, anaerobic bowel organisms)
- Cervical lesions—polyps, cancer, herpes simplex virus, warts (HPV)
- Foreign bodies (tampon, condom)
- Trauma—to vagina or cervix

In many women, especially those on the COCP or during or following pregnancy, the squamocolumnar junction is located well onto the vaginal surface of the cervix. The exposed endocervical tissue (ectopy or ectropion) is mucus-producing and may be responsible for symptomatic discharge.

You also perform a bimanual examination for Sara. The polyp is easily palpable but otherwise the uterus is normal in size, anteverted and mobile. There is no tenderness in the fornices or over the uterosacral ligaments, and no palpable masses in the adnexae.

What is your next step?

You explain your findings to Sara when she is dressed and back in your consulting room. You explain that cervical polyps with the attachment of the stalk clearly visible can be removed easily with sponge forceps in your surgery but as you cannot see the top you will refer her back to Dr Pepper for its removal at hysteroscopy (Fig. 21.1), and probably inspection of the remainder of the cervical canal and uterine cavity for further polyps.

'Could the polyp be stopping me getting pregnant?' Sara asks. *'And has it grown since my last Pap smear?'*

'Yes and yes', you answer. 'The polyp is certainly physically blocking access to the cervical canal, as well as being the undoubted cause of the discharge.

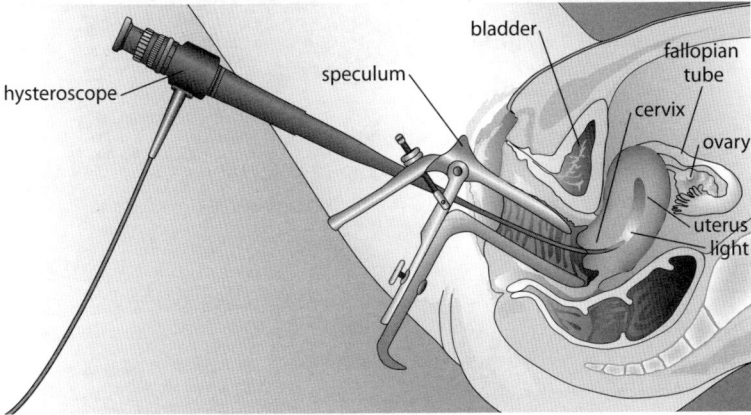

Figure 21.1 Hysteroscopy. The entire cavity of the uterus as well as the cervical canal is directly inspected during a diagnostic hysteroscopy. Using an operative hysteroscope, polyps and subserous fibroids may be resected, specimens taken directly from suspicious areas, and the endometrium ablated or excised.

The polyp consists of the same tissue that lines the canal of your cervix, tissue that produces plenty of mucus, which is what the discharge is. The polyp needs to be removed anyway, to confirm that it is benign.'

An appointment is made for Sara with Dr Pepper and you receive a letter saying that the polyp has been successfully removed. The histopathology report shows a benign endocervical polyp. No further abnormality was detected on hysteroscopy and an endometrial biopsy taken at the time shows normal secretory endometrium. Her Pap smear has also been reported as normal.

> Three months later Sara comes to see you again. 'The discharge has gone', she says, 'sex isn't a problem any more and what's more my period is a week overdue.'

You perform a urinary β-HCG for Sara, which is positive. She is delighted with this news. You make a further appointment for herself and her partner in 2 weeks time to discuss arrangements for antenatal care.

Causes of dyspareunia

Superficial (at introitus)

- Vaginal infections (e.g. candidiasis)
- Vulval infections (e.g. herpes simplex virus, HPV)
- Atrophic vaginitis—lactational or postmenopausal

Deep (within pelvis)

- Endometriosis
- Pelvic infection (acute or chronic)
- Ovarian cysts or other ovarian lesions
- Adenomyosis

Dyspareunia may be psychosexual in origin or may be exacerbated by psychological and emotional factors.

Clinical pearls

- New symptoms in a patient whose medical history is well known should not be automatically attributed to the original condition; history, examination and investigation of the presentation is always warranted.

References and further reading

Allaire C. Endometriosis and infertility: a review. J Reprod Med 2006; 51(3):164–8.

Appleyard TL, Mann CH, Khan KS. Guidelines for the management of pelvic pain associated with endometriosis: a systematic appraisal of their quality. BJOG 2006; 113(7):749–57.

Kennedy S, Bergqvist A, Chapron C et al. ESHRE guideline for the diagnosis and treatment of endometriosis. Hum Reprod 2005; 20(10):2698–704.

Royal College of Obstetricians and Gynaecologists. Clinical Green-top Guidelines: Endometriosis—Investigation and Management. Available online at www.rcog.org.uk.

Shaw RW, Souter WP, Stanton SL, eds. Gynaecology. 3rd edn. London: Churchill Livingstone, 2003:37–44, 65–66.

Part 3
Clinical Cases in Obstetrics

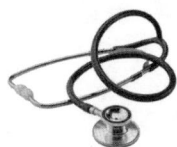

Case 22
Lucy's long labour leads to further problems …

Lucy is a 27-year-old primigravida who presents to the birth suite one Sunday morning about 7 am. She is 41 weeks pregnant and you are called to the birth suite to assess her on admission.

What is your first step?

You need to take an appropriate history. This is made easier by the fact that Lucy has been having shared care with her general practitioner, Dr Cameron, and she brings with her the shared care card (Fig. 22.1) she has been carrying. You see from this that Lucy has always enjoyed good health, having no medical or surgical history of note apart from an appendicectomy, she takes no drugs, has no allergies, her Pap smears are up to date and she has attended antenatal classes with her partner Patrick.

Further information about investigations during pregnancy is also noted on this card. Lucy's initial blood and urine tests were all within normal limits—her blood group is A Rh positive and no antibodies were detected. Throughout pregnancy her blood pressure (BP) has been in the range 110/70–120/80 mmHg, the uterine fundus has measured appropriately and fetal movements have been felt. Lucy was sure of the date of her last menstrual period, having carefully planned this pregnancy, and the dates were confirmed when Lucy had her 18-week ultrasound scan, which showed no abnormality in the fetus.

Lucy reports that she has been having mild, irregular lower abdominal pains since 10 pm the previous night, although she has been able to get some sleep. At 6 am she was awakened by a gush of fluid from her vagina and she wonders if her waters have broken. There are normal fetal movements.

What examination is made for Lucy?

Lucy's temperature, pulse rate and blood pressure are all normal and a short cardiotocograph (CTG) trace shows the fetal heart rate to have a baseline

LMP: **CYCLE:**   **AGREED EDC:**
INVESTIGATIONS: **ULTRASOUND:** Date: Weeks:
BOOKING: Date

BLOOD GROUP   ANTIBODIES   Hb   RPR   HEPB   HEPC   RUBELLA
HIV   MSU

24 – 28 WEEKS: Date   **34 – 36 WEEKS:** Date
Hb   Antibodies   Hb   Antibodies   RPR
40 WEEKS: Date
Hb   Antibodies

ANTENATAL VISITS   **DISCUSSIONS**   **Comments**

DATE	B.P.	Oedema	GEST Calc	GEST Size	Pres	1/5 Palp	Liquor Volume	F.H.S.	F.M.	Return
								Sig.		
								Sig.		
								Sig.		
								Sig.		
								Sig.		
								Sig.		
								Sig.		
								Sig.		
								Sig.		
								Sig.		
								Sig.		
								Sig.		
								Sig.		
								Sig.		

DISCUSSIONS

- ☐ Ultrasound
- ☐ Exercise
- ☐ Pelvic Floor Exercise
- ☐ Optimal Fetal Positioning
- ☐ Perineal Massage
- ☐ Signs of Labour
- ☐ When to Come In
- ☐ Hospital Access

Pain Management
- ☐ Non–Medicated
- ☐ Medicated

- ☐ 3rd Stage
- ☐ Vitamin K
- ☐ Hep B Vaccination
- ☐ Length of Stay
- ☐ EMS
- ☐ Breastfeeding

Special Requests for Birth

Figure 22.1 Shared care card for use by pregnant women

about 140 bpm with a reactive pattern. While being admitted by midwife Nerissa, Lucy has found that the contractions have become stronger, longer and more regular. Nerissa reports that Lucy is, in fact, contracting every 3 minutes, the contractions lasting 60–90 seconds. Lucy is in moderate discomfort.

What further examination do you perform for Lucy?

You inspect and palpate Lucy's abdomen. The fundal height measures 42 cm and you see that Dr Cameron has written 'big baby' on the shared care card. The presentation is cephalic with four-fifths of the head above the pelvic brim and the baby's back far out on the mother's left side. You conclude that the baby is probably lying in a left occipito-posterior position. Since Lucy appears to be in established labour you perform a vaginal examination after scrubbing and donning sterile gloves. You find that the cervix is very soft, almost completely effaced, posterior and 4 cm dilated. The forewaters are still intact, although a little fluid is draining vaginally. Through the membranes you can feel that the baby's head is loosely applied to the cervix, at a level 3 cm above the ischial spines, and you can just make out the sagittal suture line running diagonally in relation to the maternal pelvis, although you are unable to palpate either fontanelle. Your findings confirm that Lucy is in established labour and support your impression of a left occipito-posterior position.

What information do you now give to this couple?

You explain your findings to Lucy and Patrick, including the information that occipito-posterior positions are common with first babies, that sometimes this can make the labour slower as the baby's head has to rotate anteriorly through 135°, and that Lucy should consider whether she would like an epidural during labour. Lucy has been well informed about epidural analgesia during her antenatal classes but you give her an information leaflet to refresh her memory. For the moment Lucy feels able to cope with the contractions and she plans to get back under the shower to benefit from the warm water, which she found soothing. You reassure Lucy and Patrick that all is well, explain that labour will be observed but that there is no indication for any intervention at this point, and leave her in the care of Nerissa. A partogram (Fig. 22.2) is started to record and assess the progress of Lucy's labour, and warning and action lines are drawn.

....HOSPITAL

PARTOGRAM

---

1 DATE:_____ **TIME:**_____

VAGINA

CERVIX: EFFACEMENT_____

CONSISTENCY_____

DILATATION_____

APPLICATION OF P.P._____

MEMBRANES_____

LIQUOR AMNII_____

PRESENTING PART

NATURE_____

LEVEL _____

SUTURES_____

FONTANELLES_____

POSITION_____

CAPUT_____

MOULDING_____

A

R | | L

P

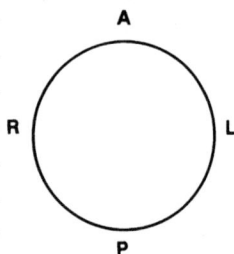

PELVIC ASSESSMENT

PROCEDURES & RECOMMENDATIONS

SIGNATURE_____

Figure 22.2 A partogram is commenced when a woman enters a birth suite and is found to have reached 4 cm cervical dilatation (the protocols may vary between different units). Warning and action lines are drawn 2 hours and

DATE		E.D.C.	GRAVID. PARITY:			
COMMENCEMENT OF CONTRACTIONS			DATE	TIME	SURNAME:	U.R. NO.
					FIRST NAMES:	
RUPTURE OF MEMBRANES	SPONTANEOUS A.R.M.		DATE	TIME		
					DOCTOR	

TIME HOURS

1 DIVISION=½hr

	190 180 170 160 150	1 2 3 4 5 6 7 8 9 10 11 12
FOETAL	140 130	
HEART	120 110	
RATE	100 90 80 70 60	

LIQUOR POSITION

C E R V I X — O / DESCENT

10 9 8 7 6 5 4 3 2 1 0

X

warning line — — — action line

OXYTOCIN (MU/MIN)

CONTRACTIONS PER 10 MINS WITH DURATION (SECS)

5 4 3 2 1

DRUGS AND I.V. FLUIDS (INC. EPIDURAL)

TEMPERATURE

BLOOD PRESSURE

MATERNAL PULSE

URINE { VOMITUS VOLUME PROTEIN ACETONE GLUCOSE }

BOWELS

1 2 3 4 5 6 7 8 9 10 11 12

4 hours respectively to the right of the projected cervical dilatation rate of 1 cm per hour. Delay in labour is suggested when the warning line is crossed and diagnosed when the action line is reached.

How is Lucy's labour monitored?

Four hours later you are requested to see Lucy again. Contractions have continued to be regular every 2–3 minutes and are moderate to strong. Initially, Lucy coped well without analgesia but 2 hours ago she asked for an injection of pethidine. This was effective for some time but now Lucy is complaining of severe back pain and requesting an epidural.

How should you proceed?

You re-examine Lucy but on abdominal palpation it is difficult to ascertain whether there has been any abdominal descent of the head because of Lucy's generalised discomfort. However, on vaginal examination you find that the cervix has changed very little since the previous examination—effacement is complete but there has been no further dilatation or rotation or descent of the head. You explain that Lucy has, in fact, crossed the action line on the partogram and you must decide on a plan of action. You tell Lucy and Patrick that you will call an anaesthetist to perform an epidural for Lucy and that you would also like to rupture the membranes (ARM). This will enable the head to be more closely applied to the cervix and bring about the production of increased amounts of natural prostaglandin. You use an amnihook to rupture the forewaters: the liquor is clear and the fetal heart following the procedure is within the normal range. At the time of ARM you also insert an indwelling urethral catheter. The anaesthetist, Dr Barry, explains the epidural procedure briefly to Lucy, who signs a consent form. Dr Barry then inserts a combined spinal-epidural anaesthetic (Fig. 22.3) and Lucy gains effective pain relief from the block. You commence Lucy on continuous electronic fetal monitoring.

Continuous electronic fetal heart rate monitoring is not used routinely in normal labour in most centres, only 'at-risk' pregnancies are continuously monitored in labour. Continuous CTG monitoring during labour is associated with a reduction in neonatal seizures, but not with significant differences in the incidence of cerebral palsy or with decreased perinatal mortality rates; furthermore continuous monitoring has been shown to be associated with increased rates of interventions including caesarean sections and operative vaginal delivery. Fetal scalp blood sampling (for pH or lactic acid measurement) used in conjunction with continuous monitoring can reduce the incidence of false-positive diagnosis of fetal distress, and hence of unnecessary intervention. Fetal ECG wave form analysis

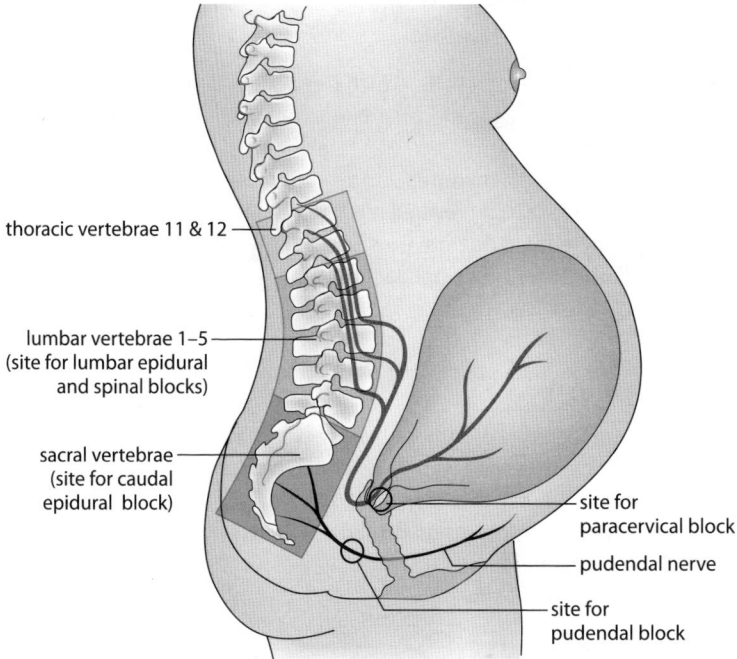

Figure 22.3 Sites for regional anaesthesia, including epidural sites

is currently being trialled for detection of fetal compromise during labour but requires an internal (scalp) electrode after membrane rupture. Indications for continuous CTG monitoring include pre-term labour, prolonged labour, suspected fetal compromise (e.g. meconium-stained liquor, fetal heart rate abnormalities noted on auscultation), the use of oxytocin infusions, epidural analgesia, previous caesarean section, multiple pregnancy and any condition that led to antenatal CTG monitoring.

About four hours later at 4 pm you come to assess Lucy again. Although tired she is quite comfortable and has been able to sleep. Abdominal palpation shows only two-fifths of the head above the brim now; vaginal examination shows the cervix to be 6 cm dilated with a well-applied head in the left transverse position 1 cm above the spines. However, Nerissa reports that contractions over the past hour have been weaker on palpation and much less frequent, about every 5–6 minutes. The CTG trace has been satisfactory throughout the previous 4 hours.

Risks of epidural analgesia

- Maternal motor blockade, which can limit or prevent movement
- Loss of bladder sensation, leading to need for urinary catheter
- Need for continuous electronic fetal monitoring
- Possible maternal hypotension
- Slight increase in the overall length of labour
- Slight increase in operative vaginal delivery rates
- Small risk of postnatal headache

What is your next step?

The partogram shows that although Lucy has made some progress she is still well to the right of the action line. You decide that Lucy's labour needs augmenting. You explain this to her and arrange an oxytocin infusion—she has already had an intravenous cannula inserted by Dr Barry when the epidural was performed.

Clinical comment

To institute an oxytocin infusion for induction or acceleration of labour, a main-line infusion of Hartmann's solution or normal saline is commenced, with a T-connector inserted between the intravenous (IV) cannula and the IV tubing; this infusion is run slowly to keep the line open. An oxytocin infusion, composed of 500 mL of Hartmann's solution containing 10 units of oxytocin, is commenced via the T-connector. The infusion rate is increased half-hourly until the desired labour pattern is achieved.

Table 22.1 Oxytocin dose achieved by infusion rate

Fluid load (mL/h)	Dose achieved (micro-units/min)
10	3.25
20	6.5
30	9.75
40	13
60	19.5
80	26.5
120	39

10 units oxytocin in 500 mL of Hartmann's solution equals 0.02 units oxytocin per mL.

What is your further management of Lucy?

At 6.30 pm you come to reassess Lucy. Another midwife, Brenda, is now caring for her and reports that contractions are regular and strong. You can see from the CTG trace (Fig. 22.4) that contractions are occurring every 2.5 minutes and that the fetal heart shows accelerations with contractions and good variability between contractions. On abdominal palpation no head can be felt; vaginal examination shows the cervix to be almost fully dilated with just an anterior lip palpable. The head has rotated to the left occipito-anterior position—you are easily able to feel the posterior fontanelle behind and to the left of the pubic symphysis—and has descended to the level of the iliac spines. You reassure Lucy that she has progressed extremely well and that vaginal delivery seems very likely. All maternal observations are satisfactory.

At 7.45 pm, while you are drinking a cup of coffee in the doctors' on-call room, you receive an urgent summons to the birth suite: 'Come immediately, the shoulders are stuck!'

What is your immediate action?

You proceed at full speed to the birth suite and find that Lucy has successfully delivered the baby's head '5 minutes ago', Brenda says. The head is still in the occipito-anterior position but there has been no external rotation. As you enter the room Lucy is pushing hard but there is no onward progress or rotation of the head. The baby's face rests on the mother's perineum, the chin is not visible and the baby is a deep blue in colour. Brenda has already called for help from other midwives who now arrive. You quickly explain to Lucy the urgency of the situation and assist Brenda to acutely flex Lucy's legs in McRoberts' manoeuvre. You direct a second midwife to feel above the pubic symphysis for the more anterior shoulder and to be ready with the next contraction to push that shoulder forward beneath the pubic arch. You send a medical student to call a paediatrician. With some difficulty you insert two fingers of your left hand into the vagina to protect the baby's face while you cut a J-shaped episiotomy on the right side of Lucy's perineum. With the next contraction you carefully grasp the baby's head over the mandibles and malar bones and with maternal effort and suprapubic pressure the anterior shoulder descends far enough for you to reach into the axilla and deliver the arm. Lifting the baby forward and up succeeds in dislodging the posterior shoulder and the remainder of the delivery takes place uneventfully. By this stage the paediatrician has arrived and takes over resuscitation of the baby, a boy. The Apgar score at 1 minute is 5 but by 5 minutes baby Jordan is crying lustily, the Apgar score is 10 and he can be handed to his proud parents.

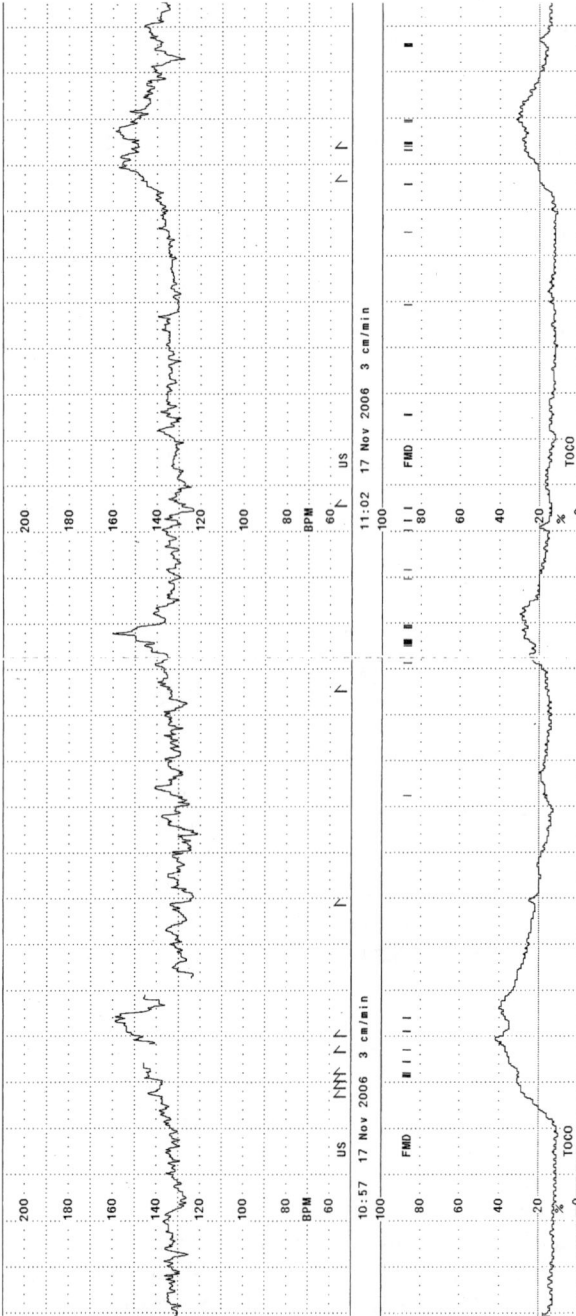

Figure 22.4 Cardiotocograph trace showing normal baseline fetal heart rate (120–160 bpm), continuous variability in fetal heart rate >15 bpm, accelerations with contractions, and no decelerations

Drill for the management of shoulder dystocia

- Call for help—more midwives, paediatrician, anaesthetist
- McRoberts' manoeuvre—abduction and acute flexion of hips by assistants
- Consider performing episiotomy (access may be difficult, may need to be midline)
- Suprapubic pressure by assistant (downward and lateral pressure to push fetal shoulder under pubic bone) to aid delivery of anterior arm
- Deliver the posterior arm after lifting baby's head anteriorly

If the above is not successful

- Roll the patient onto all fours and encourage pushing while awaiting further help
- It is important at all times to avoid fundal pressure and excessive traction or rotation attempts on the fetal head.

With some relief you deliver the placenta—placing your left hand on the abdomen you feel that separation has occurred and gentle traction on the cord is all that is required (Fig. 22.5).

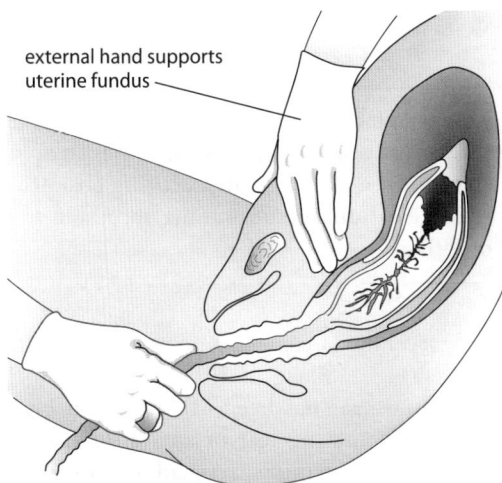

external hand supports uterine fundus

Figure 22.5 Delivery of the placenta using controlled cord traction following signs of placental separation

However, almost immediately there is a gush of bright red blood which quickly develops into a rapid haemorrhage estimated at 800 mL.

How do you manage this new development?

On palpation of the abdomen you find that the uterus is relaxed although one ampoule of oxytocin/ergometrine has been given intramuscularly once the baby was born, as is normal practice in your unit. You rub up a contraction through the abdominal wall, check that Lucy's indwelling urinary catheter is draining freely and order 40 units of oxytocin to be placed in a litre of Hartmann's solution, to be run in over 4 hours to help maintain the uterus well contracted. You collect a blood sample from Lucy for an urgent haemoglobin level and for cross-match of 2 units of packed red blood cells.

Bleeding diminishes in amount but is still excessive. Analgesia from the epidural is still very adequate so you proceed to a rapid inspection of the lower genital tract, looking for other sources of blood loss. You find that there is bleeding from several sites in your episiotomy but that this has not extended into the anorectal region, and that there is also a large anterior laceration around the clitoris and urethral meatus which, although superficial, is contributing significantly to the blood loss. You inspect the upper vagina and cervix, applying sponge forceps to the anterior and posterior cervical lips—there are no other lacerations, blood loss through the cervical os has slowed to an acceptable level and the uterus continues to be well contracted.

> 'The empty, contracted, uninjured uterus does not bleed in the presence of a normal coagulation mechanism' is an aphorism that should be remembered by everyone practising obstetrics; this can be further reduced to 'tone, tissue, trauma, thrombin' to remember the causes of PPH.

You repair the lacerations using 2/0 polyglactin and the episiotomy in anatomical layers (Fig. 22.6), again with 2/0 polyglactin. Then, having made sure that haemostasis has been achieved, you perform a rectal examination to confirm that no tear or suture extends into the rectal mucosa. You arrange with the midwifery staff to perform regular checks of the uterine fundus and of blood loss and to call you if there are further concerns, and you order a full blood count (FBC) for Lucy, to be performed the following morning.

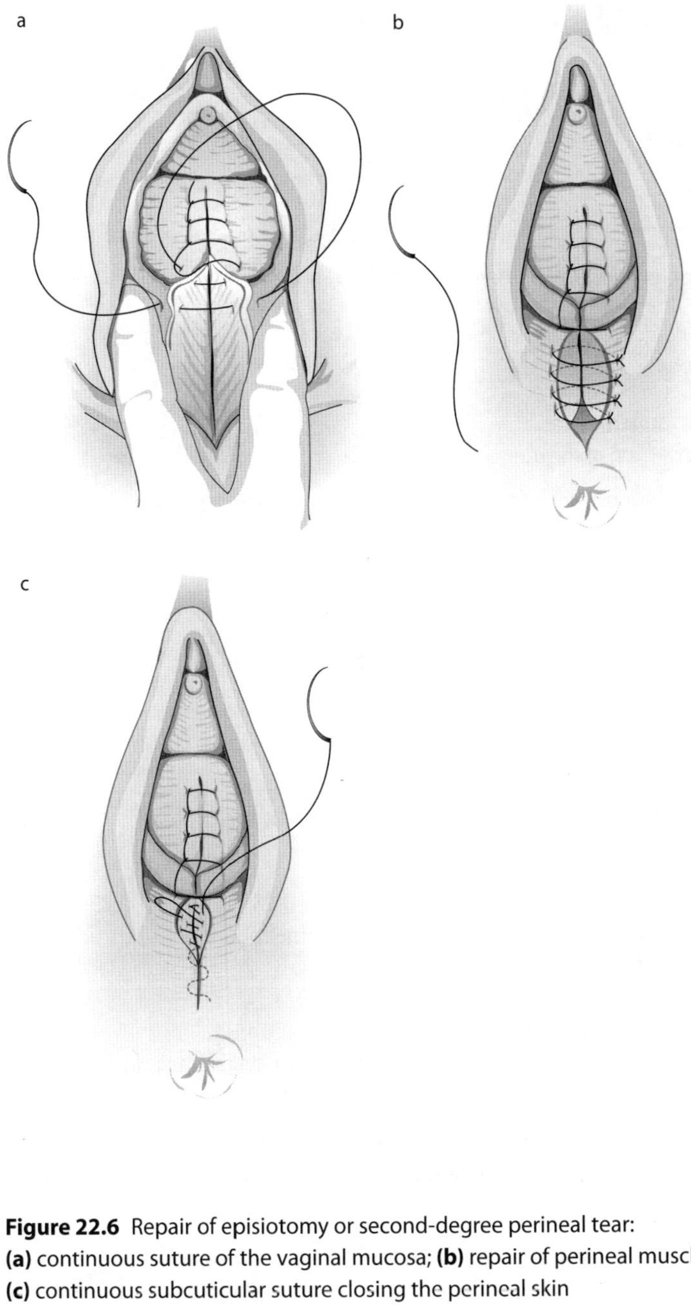

a

b

c

Figure 22.6 Repair of episiotomy or second-degree perineal tear:
(a) continuous suture of the vaginal mucosa; **(b)** repair of perineal muscles;
(c) continuous subcuticular suture closing the perineal skin

Causes of postpartum haemorrhage

Atonic uterus

- Grand multiparity
- Multiple pregnancy (overdistended uterus)
- Polyhydramnios (overdistended uterus)
- Prolonged labour
- Prior antepartum haemorrhage (e.g. placenta praevia or abruption)

Retained placenta or membranes (uterus not empty)

Genital tract trauma

- Vaginal tear
- Cervical tear
- Ruptured uterus
- Inversion of the uterus

Coagulation defects including disseminated intravascular coagulation

Clinical comment

Drill for management of postpartum haemorrhage

- Call for help
- Insert large bore (14 or 16G) IV cannula and run Hartmann's or normal saline stat
- Take blood for FBC and cross-match of 2 units of packed cells
- If the placenta is still in situ, it must be removed—manually, if necessary (under anaesthesia)
- Give a further dose of ergometrine 0.5–0.25 mg IV and 0.25 mg IM (do not give more than 1 mg ergometrine total in 24-hour period). Misoprostol 800 µg may be given orally.
- Insert urinary catheter
- Rub uterine fundus to stimulate a contraction
- Insert 40 units of oxytocin in 1 litre of normal saline and infuse at a 4–6-hourly rate

If bleeding continues at this point, you will need to conduct examination under anaesthesia. Contact theatre and anaesthetic staff. Warn the patient about the risk of laparotomy and possible hysterectomy.

- Examine the uterus under anaesthesia to exclude retained placenta or membranes.

- Examine the cervix for bleeding lacerations with two sponge-holding forceps.
- Examine the vagina for lacerations.

If still bleeding, prepare a solution of prostaglandin $F_{2\alpha}$ ($PGF_{2\alpha}$)—1 mg $PGF_{2\alpha}$ mixed with 10 mL normal saline (1 mg/mL). Inject 1 mL of this solution directly into the myometrium via the abdomen, and rub the uterine fundus. Repeat at 1-minute intervals.

- If bleeding is not controlled, the patient requires laparotomy. Cross-match more packed cells, order platelets and fresh frozen plasma, and summon specialist help. At laparotomy repair of lacerations, hysterectomy, iliac artery ligation and the B-Lynch suture compression and thereby contraction of the uterus are all possible options for controlling haemorrhage but are specialist procedures.

Clinical pearls

- When a large baby is predicted antenatally, shoulder dystocia should always be kept in mind. Everyone practising obstetrics should know the drill for shoulder dystocia thoroughly.
- A prolonged first stage of labour may herald difficulties with the second stage, requiring intervention. This may then predispose to postpartum haemorrhage, from either uterine atony or genital tract trauma.

References and further reading

Alfirevic Z, Devane D, Gyte GM. Continuous cardiotocography (CTG) as a form of electronic fetal monitoring (EFM) for fetal assessment during labour. Cochrane Database Syst Rev 2006; 3:CD006066.

Baston H. Midwifery basics: complications (6). Postpartum haemorrhage. Pract Midwife 2006; 9(4):27–31.

Creasy R, Resnik R, eds. Maternal–Fetal Medicine—Principles and Practice. 5th edn. Philadelphia: WB Saunders, 2004: 671–99.

Kwek K, Yeo GS. Shoulder dystocia and injuries: prevention and management. Curr Opin Obstet Gynecol 2006; 18(2):123–8.

Maughan KL, Heim SW, Galazka SS. Preventing postpartum hemorrhage: managing the third stage of labor. Am Fam Physician 2006; 73(6):1025–8.

Neilson JP. Fetal electrocardiogram (ECG) for fetal monitoring during labour. Cochrane Database Syst Rev 2006; 3:CD000116.

Royal College of Obstetricians and Gynaecologists. Clinical Green-top Guidelines: Shoulder Dystocia. Available online at www.rcog.org.uk.

Society of Obstetricians and Gynaecologists of Canada. Clinical Practice Guidelines: Prevention and Management of Postpartum Haemorrhage. Available online at www.socg.org.

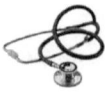

Case 23
Megan develops pre-eclampsia …

Megan is a 26-year-old primigravida you have been called to see in the day pregnancy clinic.

Megan has been having antenatal care shared between her general practitioner Dr Moore and the hospital antenatal clinic. She made her first visit to the clinic at 11 weeks' gestation, when she was booked for delivery in your hospital. She carries with her a hand-held patient record on which Dr Moore and the hospital doctors and midwives have made notes of all visits.

What is your first step in the care of Megan?

You take an appropriate history. Much of this comes from the hand-held patient record. From this you learn that Megan has no previous significant medical history apart from an appendicectomy at the age of 15. Her menarche was at age 12, and she started the combined oral contraceptive pill (COCP) at the age of 15 for dysmenorrhoea; she continued it when she became sexually active at the age of 18. This is a planned pregnancy—Megan became pregnant 3 months after stopping the pill. Her Pap smears are up to date.

Megan's booking blood pressure at 11 weeks of pregnancy was 110/70 mmHg. She experienced some mild nausea and vomiting in the first trimester but otherwise the pregnancy has been unremarkable; all blood pressures have been within the range 110/70–120/80 mmHg and until the previous day Megan has continued her work as a librarian.

Why has Megan presented to the hospital now?

Yesterday at 36 weeks' gestation in Dr Moore's surgery her blood pressure was found to be 135/90 mmHg. After resting on the couch for several minutes it was re-checked and found to be 130/85 mmHg. Megan felt perfectly well—on questioning by Dr Moore she denied any headache, abdominal pain, visual disturbance or ankle swelling, and was feeling normal fetal movements.

Examination of her abdomen showed the fundal height to measure 36 cm, the expected size for 36 weeks, the baby was in a longitudinal lie with the head presenting, and four-fifths of the fetal head was palpable above the pelvic brim. Dr Moore tested Megan's reflexes and these were not abnormally brisk, nor was any clonus present. Testing of a urine sample showed +1 of proteinuria. Dr Moore arranged for Megan to attend the day pregnancy clinic the following morning.

What are your concerns for Megan?

Your main concern is that Megan may be developing pre-eclampsia, a common condition in primigravidae in the latter weeks of pregnancy. On questioning Megan you find that she still feels quite well and the baby is moving normally. Her blood pressure is 145/90 mmHg, general physical examination is unremarkable apart from +1 ankle oedema and reflexes are normal with no clonus. Proteinuria of +1 was demonstrated on dipstick testing of the urine. A CTG is carried out and this shows a baseline fetal heart rate of 140 bpm, the trace is reactive and variable with no decelerations.

You order blood tests—FBC, electrolytes, urea and urate levels, and liver function tests (LFTs)—and a 24-hour urine collection for protein, which Megan can perform at home. You then allow Megan to go home to rest with instructions to return to the day pregnancy clinic the following day, or to telephone the birth suite if she develops headache, abdominal pain or any other symptom that concerns her overnight.

In the day pregnancy clinic the following day you find Megan's blood pressure to be 150/100 mmHg. She states she has a mild frontal headache and she feels that her ankles, fingers and face are swollen. On examination you find the reflexes to be brisker than on the previous day but there is no clonus. The CTG shows no abnormality. The results of blood tests from the previous day show that Megan's FBC, urea, creatinine, electrolytes and liver function tests are all within normal limits but her urate level is slightly raised.

What is your management plan now for Megan?

You explain to Megan that she does appear to be developing pre-eclampsia. The diagnosis depends on the result of her 24-hour urine collection but certainly her symptoms are worsening, her blood pressure is rising and it is therefore important to monitor both her wellbeing and that of her baby. You recommend hospital admission for closer observation and possible intervention in the pregnancy. She understands and agrees to this. You reassure her that with pre-eclampsia the outlook for herself and her baby is excellent but that treatment, including delivery of her baby earlier than she had anticipated, may be indicated.

Clinical comment

What is pre-eclampsia?

Pre-eclampsia is defined as hypertension with proteinuria occurring after 20 weeks' gestation. Non-dependent oedema is also usually present. There may be associated hepatic, neurological, haematological or other dysfunction.

Hypertension is defined as a systolic blood pressure ≥140 mmHg and a diastolic blood pressure ≥90 mmHg. Blood pressure should be measured in the seated position and two elevated blood pressures 4–6 hours apart are needed for the diagnosis of hypertension. Proteinuria is defined as the excretion in a 24-hour period of ≥300 mg of protein—a timed urine collection must be performed.

Non-dependent oedema—not always present—includes oedema of the face and hands; sacral and lower limb oedema may also be present.

The underlying pathophysiology of pre-eclampsia is vasoconstriction and endothelial damage leading to 'leaky vessels', intravascular fluid depletion and oedema; however, the exact cause or 'trigger' for the condition is not yet completely understood. Delivery of the baby and placenta cures the condition.

Megan is admitted to the antenatal ward. Further blood tests are taken (as previously) and the 24-hour urine result is now available—this shows 650 mg of protein excreted in 24 hours (normal upper limit is 300 mg). After 1 hour of bed rest in the ward, Megan's blood pressure settles to 140/95 mmHg.

It is decided after discussion with your consultant that Megan requires delivery for her worsening pre-eclampsia and that induction of labour should be carried out. Abdominal examination shows the head to be three-fifths above the pelvic brim. You perform a vaginal examination and find the cervix to be posterior, firm, 3 cm in length and closed, the head is at –2 cm, giving a Bishop's score of 1 (Table 23.1).

What is the significance of your findings?

It is not possible to proceed directly to artificial rupture of the membranes. Preliminary treatment with a synthetic prostaglandin is needed to ripen

Table 23.1 Bishop's scoring is used to assess the cervix for suitability for induction of labour

Score	0	1	2	3
Dilatation (cm)	0	1–2	3–4	5+
Length of cervix (cm)	3	2	1	0
Station (above or below ischial spines)	−3	−2	−1, 0	+1, +2
Consistency	Firm	Medium	Soft	
Position	Posterior	Mid	Anterior	

the cervix, making it possible to rupture the membranes at a later stage and also increasing the chances of the induction leading to effective labour and vaginal birth. You insert intravaginal dinoprostone to ripen the cervix.

Overnight Megan's blood pressure remains about 140/85–95 mmHg, her headache responds to paracetamol and a CTG shows normal fetal reactivity. The following morning your vaginal examination shows the cervix to be favourable enough for artificial rupture of the membranes (ARM) to be performed (soft, 1 cm in length, mid-position, 2 cm dilated, at spines, Bishop score 2). An oxytocin infusion is commenced. Blood tests are repeated—the results are similar to the previous occasion, in particular, Megan has a platelet count of 290×10^9/L, confirming her suitability for epidural anaesthesia. Her blood pressure at this time is 140/95 mmHg. Megan's partner Brad is present in the birth suite to support her.

How should Megan's labour be managed?

Megan will be under close observation by both the midwifery and the medical staff. Regular contractions begin within 4 hours. At this time Megan's blood pressure is noted to be 150/100 mmHg, and an epidural catheter is inserted by an anaesthetist. The blood pressure settles to 120/80 mmHg but within 1 hour has risen again to 170/110 mmHg. A urinary catheter is also inserted at this time and Megan's urine output, measured hourly, remains >30 mL per hour.

What are your immediate concerns and how do you deal with these?

Megan's pre-eclampsia is worsening and you are concerned about the possibility of a seizure; you are also concerned about the development of renal and liver complications. Megan is transferred to the high dependency area of the birth suite where hydralazine and magnesium sulfate infusions are started. Further blood tests are ordered urgently—these show elevated urate levels of 0.55 mmol/L, but a normal platelet count at 266×10^9/L. The oxytocin infusion is continued, and Megan's contractions are regular every 3 minutes, lasting 60–90 seconds. However, her blood pressure is difficult to control, with increasing levels of hydralazine needed to keep it at 160/110 mmHg, and 4 hours after inserting the epidural your vaginal examination shows the cervix to be only 3 cm dilated.

Not all maternity units will have a high dependency area but most will have at least one separate room for the management and one-to-one nursing of high-risk cases.

The complications of severe pre-eclampsia

- Renal—decreased glomerular filtration rate, proteinuria, oliguria, renal failure
- Haematological and vascular—thrombocytopenia, coagulopathy, microangiopathic anaemia, severe hypertension (>170/110 mmHg)
- Neurological—headache, visual disturbance, hyperreflexia, seizures (eclampsia), cerebrovascular accident, blindness
- Pulmonary—pulmonary oedema
- Hepatic—raised liver enzymes, subcapsular haematoma, hepatic rupture
- Fetal—retarded intrauterine growth, oligohydramnios, placental abruption, fetal hypoxia, fetal death
- HELLP syndrome—occurs in 20% of women with severe pre-eclampsia

---

HELLP syndrome (Haemolysis—haemolytic microangiopathic anaemia, Elevated Liver enzymes, Low Platelets) indicates rapid deterioration in the woman's condition and the need for urgent delivery.

Clinical comment

Control of blood pressure in severe pre-eclampsia

Aim to keep the blood pressure in the range 140/90–160/100 mmHg—at blood pressures ≥170/110 mmHg there is a significant risk of cerebral haemorrhage, at blood pressures below a diastolic of 90 mmHg placental perfusion may be compromised, resulting in fetal distress. Continuous CTG monitoring is essential.

An antihypertensive should be administered parenterally. The most widely used is hydralazine 5–10 mg given by slow IV injection followed by an IV infusion; 80 mg hydralazine is diluted to 40 mL with normal saline and administered by syringe pump, commencing at 1 mL per hour. The rate of infusion is titrated against the blood pressure and the maximum dose should not exceed 30 mL per hour (60 mg per hour). If the maternal pulse rises above 100 bpm, a beta-blocker may be used; alternatively hydralazine should be ceased and other antihypertensives started. Metoprolol and nifedipine have all been extensively used in this situation; however, it should be noted that difficulty controlling blood pressure usually indicates urgent need for delivery.

Patients with severe pre-eclampsia are usually but not always hypovolaemic and hypoalbuminaemic, with resulting oliguria. A urinary catheter should be inserted and output measured hourly. Colloid solutions should be given cautiously intravenously in boluses rather than increasing the infusion rate, with careful monitoring to avoid pulmonary oedema. In difficult cases a central venous pressure (CVP) line should be inserted and fluid replaced to maintain a pressure of 8 mmHg and urine output of ≥30 mL per hour. Iatrogenic fluid overload and pulmonary oedema must be avoided.

What is appropriate management for Megan at this point?

In view of Megan's deteriorating pre-eclampsia a decision is made by your consultant for caesarean section. You explain this decision to Megan and Brad. Since you have already clearly explained to them everything that has happened to Megan since her admission, they understand the situation, the fact that Megan's high blood pressure endangers both herself and the baby, and that caesarean section is strongly indicated medically. Brad will accompany Megan to the operating theatre and Megan will have the operation performed under epidural. The anaesthetist comes to institute this arrangement.

The decision–incision interval is just under 1 hour. You assist at the caesarean section, which results in the delivery of a baby girl. The baby is in good condition, with Apgar scores of 8 at 1 minute and 10 at 5 minutes, and Megan and Brad are able to hold her very soon after birth.

How do you manage Megan postoperatively?

Following the caesarean section, Megan's blood pressure stabilises at 140/90 mmHg but Megan remains in the high dependency unit for 24 hours on magnesium sulfate and hydralazine as her reflexes remain brisk and it is well recognised that eclampsia can occur postpartum. Gradually her condition returns to normal.

Clinical comment

Anticonvulsant therapy in severe pre-eclampsia

Magnesium sulfate 50% is the prophylactic anticonvulsant drug of choice. It is administered intravenously via a syringe pump and a peripheral line—it should not be given directly via a CVP line because sudden boluses can cause marked side effects. A 4 g loading dose (8 mL) is given over 20 minutes. The maintenance dose is 1–2 g or 2–4 mL per hour. Women should be warned of possible transient hot flushes.

Magnesium may cause muscular weakness, respiratory depression and cardiac arrhythmias, and levels of magnesium may rise with poor urinary output. Respiratory rate and urine output should be monitored hourly. Patellar reflexes should be tested 4 hourly, lung bases auscultated and the jugular venous pressure checked for signs of cardiac failure. If urine output falls, there are absent reflexes, respiratory rate falls below 10 breaths/min or eclampsia supervenes then serum magnesium levels should be monitored—1.7–3.5 mmol/L is considered therapeutic. Calcium gluconate 1 g or calcium chloride (5 mL 10% solution) can help reduce magnesium levels if toxicity occurs.

Does Megan require further postnatal follow-up?

Yes. Megan is transferred to the postnatal ward on day 2, her blood pressure settles rapidly, breastfeeding is established and Megan's postnatal course is

Management of eclampsia (seizures)

- Protect the patient from harm—put up cot sides to bed, use pillows
- Secure airway—place patient on left side in coma position, insert airway
- Administer oxygen
- Obtain intravenous access if not already in place
- Use the loading dose of magnesium sulfate to control fit—diazepam has been associated with an increased maternal mortality rate
- Institute magnesium sulfate IV as outlined for the treatment of severe pre-eclampsia
- Institute hydralazine therapy as for severe pre-eclampsia
- If patient is undelivered, arrange delivery once situation stabilised

otherwise uncomplicated. She is discharged home on day 6 to have home visits from the domiciliary midwifery service of the hospital.

It is important that underlying hypertension be excluded so 6 weeks later you see Megan in the outpatients' department. She is quite well, the abdominal incision is well healed and her blood pressure is 110/70 mmHg. Breastfeeding is well established. You order an FBC, urea, electrolytes and uric acid, and all results are within normal levels. You reassure Megan that she will suffer no lasting effects of her pre-eclampsia, that she has a 50% chance of experiencing pre-eclampsia in a future pregnancy and that since the indication for the caesarean section was confined to that pregnancy she could anticipate a vaginal birth in her next pregnancy if she so wished.

Clinical pearls

- Severe pre-eclampsia requires stabilisation of blood pressure and anticonvulsant therapy followed by delivery of the baby, as the condition will not improve until after delivery, and severe pre-eclampsia threatens the lives of mother and baby.
- Women with no underlying predisposing condition who experience pre-eclampsia in a first or subsequent pregnancy have a 50% chance of a recurrence in a later pregnancy; however, the condition does not generally worsen with successive pregnancies.

References and further reading

Altman D, Carroli G, Duley L et al. Do women with pre-eclampsia, and their babies, benefit from magnesium sulphate? The Magpie Trial: a randomised placebo-controlled trial. Lancet 2002; 359(9321):1877–90.

Chamberlain G, Steer P, eds. Turnbull's Obstetrics. 3rd edn. London: Churchill Livingstone, 2001: 333–50.

Duley L, Gülmezoglu AM, Henderson-Smart DJ. Magnesium sulphate and other anticonvulsants for women with pre-eclampsia. Cochrane Database Syst Rev 2006; 3:CD000025.

Royal College of Obstetricians and Gynaecologists. Clinical Green-top Guidelines: The Management of Severe Pre-eclampsia/Eclampsia; revised March 2006. National Evidence-Based Clinical Guidelines: Electronic Fetal Monitoring, 2001. Available online at www.rcog.org.uk.

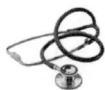

Case 24
Helen presents with raised blood pressure in pregnancy …

Helen is a 32-year-old gravida whom you have been asked to see in the antenatal clinic. She is currently 34 weeks pregnant.

Helen has had two previous vaginal deliveries and a miscarriage at 8 weeks of pregnancy. Her children are now aged 8 and 10. Since her last delivery Helen has been divorced and has re-partnered; this baby will be the first child for her partner Steve.

Helen suffers from essential hypertension. When she is not pregnant her blood pressure is well controlled with the angiotensin-converting enzyme (ACE) inhibitor monopril.

Helen has carefully planned this pregnancy knowing the implications of her hypertension and the treatment she is usually on. She had a levonorgestrel-releasing intrauterine contraceptive device (IUCD) in place for 5 years; at the time this was removed to enable her to try to conceive, which she did within 2 months, her general practitioner changed her from monopril to methyldopa, on a dose of 250 mg three times daily. Helen also commenced on folic acid supplements.

Clinical comment

Classification of hypertensive disorders in pregnancy

- Chronic hypertension—blood pressure of 140/90 mmHg or greater before pregnancy or before 20 weeks' gestation—may be essential (90% cases) or secondary to renal, endocrine or other disease
- Gestational hypertension—blood pressure of 140/90 mmHg or greater without proteinuria after 20 weeks' gestation; the diagnosis may also be made when a patient has a rise of 30 mmHg systolic, or 15 mmHg diastolic, above the known pre-pregnancy or early pregnancy blood pressure

- Pre-eclampsia—hypertension with proteinuria occurring after 20 weeks' gestation
- Eclampsia—seizure disorder following on pre-eclampsia—onset of pre-eclampsia and seizure(s) may be very sudden
- Pre-eclampsia superimposed on chronic hypertension—symptoms and/or signs of pre-eclampsia occurring after 20 weeks' gestation in a woman known to have chronic hypertension

What do you need to know about Helen's previous pregnancies?

Helen's first pregnancy was complicated by moderate pre-eclampsia superimposed on her known chronic hypertension. She required increasing doses of methyldopa to control her blood pressure and at 34 weeks developed some proteinuria and non-dependent oedema. There was a degree of intrauterine growth retardation of the fetus, which led to having labour induced at 37 weeks' gestation. The baby, a boy, weighed 2240 g and spent 4 days in the special care baby unit (SCBU) having jaundice treated.

In her second pregnancy Helen experienced some hypertension again, requiring increased methyldopa from 30 weeks. She was also treated with low-dose aspirin from 8 weeks' gestation. She did not develop proteinuria during the pregnancy; however, there was slowing of fetal growth from 32 weeks that led to the induction of labour at 38 weeks' gestation. The baby, a girl, weighed 2500 g and required treatment for jaundice in the SCBU.

How has this pregnancy been managed?

In this pregnancy Helen was first seen at the antenatal clinic at 8 weeks of pregnancy. Apart from some mild nausea she was feeling well. Her blood pressure at this time was 125/85 mmHg, which was 'good' for her, she said. She was then on methyldopa 750 mg daily. Her last Pap smear had been 10 months previously.

In addition to routine antenatal blood tests Helen had baseline urea, electrolytes and uric acid performed. Results of these were all within the normal range. She also underwent a 24-hour urine collection for total protein—the result of this was 183 mg of protein excreted in 24 hours, well within the normal range. She had a portable ultrasound scan performed to confirm her due date—she gave the date of her last menstrual period as 'certain' and had a 28-day cycle. Ultrasound showed a single fetus with a crown–rump length (CRL) of 1.5 cm as expected for 8 weeks and 2 days.

Following her last pregnancy Helen underwent full thrombophilia screening; all tests were negative. However, in view of her history of pre-eclampsia superimposed on hypertension in her first pregnancy, and intrauterine growth restriction in both previous pregnancies, Helen was commenced on low-dose aspirin (150 mg daily) at the booking visit and has continued with this throughout the pregnancy.

What are your current concerns?

On looking through Helen's notes you see that her blood pressure has been well controlled, in a range of 120/85–140/95 mmHg, during her pregnancy. Fetal growth has been assessed with ultrasound at 18 weeks, 28 weeks and 32 weeks of pregnancy. All parameters are within the 95th percentile and the baby is growing well and symmetrically; estimated fetal weight at 32 weeks was 1900 g, there was adequate liquor around the baby and Doppler studies showed systolic/diastolic (S/D) ratios of 2.9 (normal for 34 weeks).

What examination do you make for Helen?

You take Helen's blood pressure and find it to be 150/100 mmHg. On questioning, Helen feels well, with no headache or abdominal pain, and the baby is moving normally, but she is aware of some puffiness of fingers and feet, which you confirm on examination. Examination of the abdomen shows the baby to be lying longitudinally with the head presenting; the uterine fundus measures 34 cm.

You ask Helen to move into the day pregnancy unit where blood is taken for routine tests and a CTG performed. After resting for 30 minutes Helen's blood pressure is again checked and found to be 140/90 mmHg. Dipstick testing of urine shows +1 protein. Arrangements are made for Helen to perform a 24-hour urine collection for proteinuria and she is allowed to go home to return to the day pregnancy unit in 2 days' time.

> Day pregnancy units provide care for women who need assessment of pregnancy more often than regular antenatal clinics provide, but who do not need to be inpatients in hospital. They provide assessment and surveillance of women with mild-to-moderate degrees of hypertension, those with diabetes both preceding pregnancy and gestational, women with prolonged pregnancy and those with certain other complications of pregnancy. Day pregnancy units provide a particularly suitable environment for women found to have

raised blood pressure during pregnancy—the blood pressure can be checked again after a period of rest, a CTG performed and blood and urine tests arranged. In a day pregnancy unit the opportunity can be taken by staff to discuss concerns such as contraception, sterilisation, domestic violence and depression. This is often more easily done in this environment than in the context of a busy antenatal clinic.

What are your conclusions and what plans do you make for Helen?

You make a presumptive diagnosis of mild pre-eclampsia superimposed on chronic hypertension. You note that Helen has a new partner and therefore is at renewed risk of pre-eclampsia in this pregnancy. You recall that pre-eclampsia is more common in women who have pre-existing hypertension. You plan to manage Helen's condition with visits to the day pregnancy unit three times weekly to check her blood pressure, blood results, proteinuria, fetal movements and perform a CTG. You organise a further ultrasound scan to assess fetal growth, the amniotic fluid index and umbilical blood flow and arrange to review the results of this at the day pregnancy unit in 2 days' time. Your plan is to manage Helen's pregnancy expectantly unless her pre-eclampsia worsens or the baby shows signs of intrauterine growth slowing down or an abnormal CTG. You explain to Helen that expectant management will be continued to 37–38 weeks depending on her progress, and that at that stage induction of labour will probably be advised. Helen is happy with this plan, which reflects her management in her two earlier pregnancies.

Clinical pearls

- Pre-eclampsia is more common in nulliparae or in women pregnant with a new partner, diabetic women, women with multiple pregnancies or molar pregnancy, and women with chronic hypertension, renal disease, thrombophilias and connective tissue disorders.
- Expectant management of mild pre-eclampsia includes surveillance of both mother and baby—intrauterine growth retardation may occur.
- Antihypertensive therapy in mild or moderate pre-eclampsia does not modify the course of the disease and has no role.

References and further reading

Duley L, Meher S, Abalos E. Management of pre-eclampsia. BMJ 2006; 332(7539):463–8.

Meher S, Duley L. Exercise or other physical activity for preventing pre-eclampsia and its complications. Cochrane Database Syst Rev 2006; 2:CD005942.

Meher S, Duley L. Rest during pregnancy for preventing pre-eclampsia and its complications in women with normal blood pressure. Cochrane Database Syst Rev 2006; 2:CD005939.

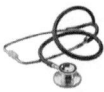

Case 25
Stacey presents to the birth suite at 28 weeks of pregnancy ...

Stacey is a 20-year-old primigravida at 28 weeks' gestation whom you meet for the first time at 3 am in the birth suite. Stacey gives a history of painful contractions every 10 minutes.

What further history do you take from Stacey?

You need to know the earlier details of Stacey's pregnancy. You also need to know whether there is any evidence of ruptured membranes associated with her contractions, and whether there has been vaginal bleeding. Stacey denies both these things. She was woken up at midnight by the painful contractions, which are now 10 minutes apart. She has had an uncomplicated pregnancy so far and her general medical history is unremarkable.

What examination do you make for Stacey?

You need to establish whether Stacey is in labour or imminently so, and determine whether there is evidence of infection. You also need to know the lie and presentation of the fetus.

Stacey is afebrile, her pulse rate is 80 bpm and her blood pressure is 120/65 mmHg. The fundal height is 28 cm, the fetal lie is longitudinal but you are unable to confirm the presentation on palpation. A bedside ultrasound examination demonstrates a cephalic presentation. The midwife Rhonda tells you that she can palpate moderately strong contractions, which appear to be increasing in intensity. The CTG is normal, with no evidence of fetal distress. You perform a speculum examination and the membranes are intact. The cervix appears slightly open and on digital examination you find the cervix 3 cm dilated and only 1 cm thick.

What do you conclude from your findings?

Stacey does appear to be in preterm labour.

Speculum examination should be performed with full aseptic technique, avoiding contact of the cervix with the speculum. Cervical swabs should be taken for immediate bacteriological assessment. If the cervix is closed and there is no blood or amniotic fluid to be seen in the vagina, a fetal fibronectin (fFN) test should be performed. Digital examination should be avoided unless there is a significant possibility of a cord presentation or prolapse.

Clinical comment

- Ten per cent of babies are born at less than 37 weeks' gestation, but only 1% are born at less than 28 weeks' gestation. These very preterm infants have high perinatal mortality and morbidity.
- There are many causes of preterm labour. The most common recognisable causes are preterm rupture of membranes, chorioamnionitis and urinary tract infection (particularly pyelonephritis). However, the pathogenesis of most cases is unknown.
- 'Threatened' preterm labour (TPL) is common. TPL implies contractions that do not lead to labour (i.e. cervical effacement and dilatation). It can be difficult to distinguish between true preterm labour and TPL. Serial cervical examinations may be necessary. Some units use an fFn test to help distinguish between these two clinical entities. Fetal fibronectin is a glycoprotein released from the decidua which is normally not detectable until term. A positive test does not mean that preterm labour is inevitable, but a negative test means it is unlikely. In other words, this test is useful because it has a good negative predictive value.

What is your immediate management of Stacey?

You explain the diagnosis of preterm labour and its treatment to Stacey. You further explain that attempts will be made to suppress her labour in order to delay delivery of the fetus for at least 48 hours while steroids are given to accelerate fetal lung maturation and while transport is arranged for her to a tertiary hospital with appropriate neonatal care facilities. The best results for the baby, you tell her, follow transfer of the baby in utero and birth in a tertiary centre, rather than postnatal transfer. You also explain that long-term results for preterm babies born at or after 28 weeks are good, both in terms of survival and in regard to long-term physical and intellectual abnormalities.

Stacey is treated with an oral nifedipine regimen to try to stop her contractions, and with betamethasone 11.4 mg IM to assist with fetal lung maturation. In fact, contractions cease over the next hour and you arrange for Stacey to be transferred to the nearest hospital with a tertiary neonatal intensive care service.

Clinical comment

- The main aim of tocolysis (stopping uterine contractions) is to allow the administration of maternal steroids, which improve fetal lung maturation and outcome. Therefore, tocolysis is only used for up to 48 hours. The effectiveness of tocolytics is difficult to assess—women who do not deliver may not have been in true preterm labour. In order not to miss true preterm labour, many women are treated who in retrospect were clearly not in preterm labour; making the diagnosis can be difficult.
- Maternal anxiety often causes difficulty with diagnosis.
- There are many drugs that can be used for tocolysis. All are similarly effective, and most have significant fetal or maternal side effects. These drugs include indomethacin, which can be administered as a suppository and is suitable for use if maternal transfer is required. It does reduce fetal renal and cerebral blood flow, and can close the ductus arteriosus in utero after 34 weeks, so this drug is not favoured by neonatologists. An oral nifedipine regimen has no fetal side effects but can cause maternal hypotension, so careful maternal observation is mandatory. Older drugs include intravenous salbutamol, which has the potential to cause serious maternal side effects, such as ketoacidosis and pulmonary oedema.
- The administration of a course of maternal steroids such as betamethasone or dexamethasone (both of these steroids cross the placenta) has been shown to reduce the incidence of fetal respiratory distress (hyaline membrane disease) and the length of time of ventilation in a neonatal intensive care unit. There is no reduction in neonatal mortality, but morbidity has been shown to be reduced when steroids are used under 34 weeks' gestation. A course of betamethasone consists of two IM doses of 11.4 mg given 24 hours apart.
- Tocolysis is contraindicated in the presence of obvious infection or significant antepartum haemorrhage.

Nifedipine administration

- Nifedipine is given as an initial dose of two 20-mg tablets. The first tablet should be chewed and taken with orange juice.
- Onset of tocolysis is within 30–60 minutes and institution of a second tocolytic should not be considered before that time.
- Minor side effects include facial flushing, headache, nausea, tachycardia and dizziness.

It is important that Stacey delivers in a hospital with tertiary neonatal intensive care facilities. Outcomes for babies are not so favourable if they have to be transferred after birth, although sometimes this is unavoidable. Certainly, a woman in active labour must not be transferred because delivery of a preterm infant en route in an ambulance or aircraft has a poorer outcome than delivering in any hospital.

Follow-up

Stacey is successfully transferred by road ambulance to the tertiary centre and you are contacted by the registrar on call the following day about her progress. Stacey has recommenced in labour; she has progressed slowly and delivered a live female infant weighing 1200 g in good condition, not requiring ventilation.

Clinical pearls

- Maternal anxiety can make diagnosis of preterm labour difficult. A calm, clear explanation about how preterm labour is managed and the probable outcomes for the baby, by allaying anxiety, can assist with both diagnosis and management.
- Significant sepsis or antepartum haemorrhage in conjunction with threatened or definite preterm labour are absolute contraindications to tocolysis and steroid administration. Urgent delivery is required regardless of the period of gestation.

References and further reading

Chamberlain G, Steer P, eds. Turnbull's Obstetrics. 3rd edn. London: Churchill Livingstone, 2001: 493–511.

Creasy R, Resnik R, eds. Maternal–Fetal Medicine—Principles and Practice. 5th edn. Philadelphia: WB Saunders, 2004: 663–8.

Groom KM, Liu E, Allenby K. The impact of fetal fibronectin testing for women with symptoms of preterm labour in routine clinical practice within a New Zealand population. Aust N Z J Obstet Gynaecol 2006; 46(5):440–5.

Roberts D, Dalziel S. Antenatal corticosteroids for accelerating fetal lung maturation for women at risk of preterm birth. Cochrane Database Syst Rev 2006; 3:CD004454.

Royal College of Obstetricians and Gynaecologists. Clinical Green-top Guidelines: Tocolytic Drugs for Women in Pre-Term Labour. Available online at www.rcog.org.uk.

Society of Obstetricians and Gynaecologists of Canada. Clinical Practice Guidelines: Antenatal Corticosteroid Therapy for Fetal Maturation. Available online at www.sogc.org.

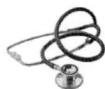

Case 26
Bronwyn is bleeding at 31 weeks of pregnancy ...

Bronwyn is a 34-year-old multipara whom you are called to see in the birth suite one Sunday afternoon. Bronwyn is gravida 5, para 5, and is at just 31 weeks' gestation in this pregnancy. She has had one set of twins born by caesarean section and has had one spontaneous vaginal birth since the caesarean. She presents with the history of a painless vaginal bleed about an hour previously. She lost about half a cup of blood, which she describes as 'running down my legs, like my waters had broken'.

What are your immediate concerns?

You must quickly establish what Bronwyn's overall status is, and whether the bleeding is continuing—antepartum haemorrhage can be swift and catastrophic. You also need some basic information about this and previous pregnancies.

Bronwyn's blood pressure is 120/70 mmHg, her pulse rate is 85 bpm and she is afebrile. You insert an intravenous cannula and draw blood for an FBC, and group and hold for blood group confirmation and cross-matching, while continuing to take her history.

Bronwyn has been having shared antenatal care with her general practitioner Dr Murray and brings her hand-held patient record. At 18 weeks she had a morphology ultrasound scan which showed a 'low-lying' placenta—she is booked for a further scan to determine the placental site at 32 weeks. Otherwise this pregnancy has been uneventful. The bleeding was not postcoital and Bronwyn has not experienced any contractions in association with the bleeding. In the past she has had three normal pregnancies ending in normal deliveries plus the caesarean section for the twins, who were both breech presentations. All her children are alive and well.

> Although about 20% of pregnancies will be noted to have a 'low-lying' placenta at 18 weeks, in 99% of women uterine growth and the formation of the lower uterine segment means that by term these placentas are normally sited.

What further examination of Bronwyn do you now carry out?

General examination shows no signs of anaemia. Bronwyn's heart and lungs appear normal.

Inspection of the abdomen shows an obvious pregnancy and a central linea nigra. There are also some striae from previous pregnancies and a Pfannenstiel scar. Palpation of the abdomen reveals a non-tender uterus measuring 33 cm in height from the top of the pubic symphysis. The uterus is soft and the fetus easily palpable, lying slightly obliquely with the head in the left iliac fossa. A CTG trace shows the fetal heart to have a baseline of 140 bpm, good reactivity and no decelerations.

Do you now perform a vaginal examination?

No! History and abdominal examination are pointing towards a diagnosis of placenta praevia; if this is the case, vaginal examination could further dislodge the placenta, causing major haemorrhage. You should inspect the vulval region and any pads used to try to assess the degree of haemorrhage but vaginal examination must not be performed.

> Do not perform vaginal examination in any case of antepartum haemorrhage until you are certain that the placenta is not praevia!

What investigations can be safely performed?

In the birth suite you perform an abdominal ultrasound using a portable machine. You obtain a reasonable view of the placenta, which lies below the fetal head and across the cervix. You explain this finding to Bronwyn and the need to admit her to hospital. Bleeding appears to have settled down but you order a cross-match of two units of blood to be kept available in view of the diagnosis. You also initiate a course of steroid injections (betamethasone 11.4 mg given twice at an interval of 24 hours) to increase surfactant production in the fetal lungs in case further bleeding necessitates urgent preterm delivery.

The following day a formal ultrasound scan is performed in the medical imaging department. It shows that the placenta lies both anteriorly and posteriorly and directly across the cervix—a central placenta praevia. There is no evidence of placenta accreta in association with the scar of the previous caesarean section. The fetus has measurements consistent with normal growth, there is adequate liquor and Doppler scans show normal umbilical blood flow.

> Placenta praevia is more common in women of higher parity and following previous caesarean section; when an anterior placenta praevia occurs in association with a prior caesarean scar, there is an increased risk of the placenta being morbidly adherent to the uterus—placenta praevia accreta. This is a very serious condition with up to 10% maternal mortality in some series.

What arrangements are now made for Bronwyn?

You explain to Bronwyn that the placenta blocks the passage of the baby to the outside world and that the only safe way of delivering her baby is by repeat caesarean section. There has been no further vaginal bleeding overnight, all Bronwyn's observations are satisfactory and the fetal heart trace is reactive. It is decided that if there is no further bleeding over the next 24 hours, then Bronwyn may be able to return to her home, which is less than 1 km from the hospital, provided that she always has access to transport if she has further bleeding and that cross-matched blood is kept available on a weekly basis.

However, overnight Bronwyn has a further small bleed and although this also settles it is decided that she must remain as an inpatient. While it is hoped that this can be until the fetus is close to term, 37–38 weeks, she understands that it may be necessary to perform urgent caesarean section at any time if a major haemorrhage occurs.

For several weeks the pregnancy continues uneventfully and Bronwyn remains in hospital. At 34 weeks there is a further moderate bleed but this also settles. Growth ultrasound scans show the baby to be growing normally. A date is selected at 37 weeks' gestation for a planned caesarean section—this is in the first week of January. Bronwyn has to face spending Christmas in hospital.

'What about tubal ligation at the time of the caesarean section?'
Bronwyn asks

Tubal ligation at the time of a caesarean section, especially a repeat caesarean, is an excellent option when the woman, and her partner, have time to discuss the matter and are aware of the advantages and disadvantages of the procedure. The risks of the procedure to the woman, over and above the risks of the caesarean surgery, are minimal, whereas the alternative procedure, laparoscopic sterilisation after an interval postnatally, carries small but nevertheless significant risks. However, the failure rate of tubal ligation is higher if it is performed at caesarean section—approximately 0.5–1 per 200 women. For Bronwyn, it is important to emphasise that placenta praevia carries risks to both mother and baby—if she were to have a tubal ligation and then experience the death of the baby in the postnatal period she may have major regrets at having decided to have the procedure done. After careful thought and discussion with her husband Bronwyn decides to have the procedure done and completes the consent forms so that it can be carried out even if an emergency caesarean is required.

You have also carefully discussed the forthcoming caesarean section with Bronwyn and completed consent forms. You have explained that she may need a blood transfusion intra- or postoperatively and that there is a small risk of her requiring a hysterectomy if there is difficulty controlling bleeding postoperatively.

At 36 weeks' gestation on Christmas Eve you are called urgently to see Bronwyn, who is experiencing a major haemorrhage. What is your immediate course of action?

You establish intravenous access and order four units of blood to be available in total. You inform your consultant and the anaesthetic team. A decision is made to proceed to an urgent caesarean section under general anaesthesia. You arrange the operation with theatre staff and inform Bronwyn's family.

You assist your consultant with a repeat lower segment caesarean section and bilateral tubal ligation. Measured blood loss during the operation is 1600 mL and Bronwyn is given a 4-unit blood transfusion. At the conclusion of the procedure vaginal bleeding has diminished and the uterus is well contracted but you arrange for Bronwyn to be observed overnight in the high dependency unit of the birth suite. The baby, a girl, has Apgar scores of 4 at 1 minute and 9 at 5 minutes, weighs 2400 g and after spending the night under observation in the special care baby unit is transferred back to her mother on Christmas Day.

> Antepartum haemorrhage due to placenta praevia may be followed by postpartum haemorrhage as the lower uterine segment being thinner than the upper myometrium contracts down less well following delivery.

Clinical pearls

- Placenta praevia is distinguished clinically from the second main cause of antepartum haemorrhage, placental abruption, by its generally painless presentation.
- A small antepartum haemorrhage may herald a catastrophic haemorrhage. Women presenting with antepartum haemorrhage require an immediate assessment in a unit in which both ultrasound scans and caesarean section can be performed and where blood bank facilities are available; women in remote areas should be transferred to an appropriate hospital setting as soon as possible.

References and further reading

Nardin JM, Kulier R, Boulvain M. Techniques for the interruption of tubal patency for female sterilisation. Cochrane Database Syst Rev 2006; 3:CD003034.

Oyelese Y, Smulian JC. Placenta previa, placenta accreta, and vasa previa. Obstet Gynecol 2006; 107(4):927–41.

Royal College of Obstetricians and Gynaecologists. Clinical Green-top Guidelines: Placenta Praevia and Placenta Praevia Accreta: Diagnosis and Management. Available online at www.rcog.org.uk.

Santoso JT, Saunders BA, Grosshart K. Massive blood loss and transfusion in obstetrics and gynecology. Obstet Gynecol Surv 2005; 60(12):827–37.

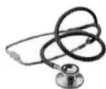

Case 27
Dora develops diabetes in pregnancy …

Dora has presented to you in the antenatal clinic for a visit at 28 weeks' gestation. Dora was born in the Philippines and her first baby was also born there, a boy who was delivered with forceps after a 26-hour labour and weighing 4300 g. Dora did not have glucose tolerance testing (GTT) in that pregnancy but in the current pregnancy, her second, because of the size of her previous child and her ethnic background, she qualifies for testing and has had a 75-g GTT the day prior to her visit. This has shown a fasting blood glucose level of 5.9 mmol/L and a 2-hour level of 9.1 mmol/L, which means that Dora has gestational diabetes mellitus (GDM).

Clinical comment

Selection of patients for GTT may be on the basis of a 50-g or 75-g glucose tolerance screening test, in which all women attending antenatal clinic are given the glucose load (non-fasting) and their blood sugar level or blood glucose level (BSL) (performed on venous blood) is measured 1 hour later; cut-off points for the two doses are 7.8 and 8.0 mmol/L respectively. Alternatively, where resources are limited or in areas of low incidence, selective screening based on recognised risk factors may be appropriate. Risk factors include a family history of diabetes, previous gestational diabetes, history of a large baby (>4200 g) or unexplained stillbirth in a previous pregnancy, multiple pregnancy, high parity, advanced maternal age, obesity and membership of certain ethnic groups, including women of South-East Asian, and Aboriginal and Torres Strait Islander background. Testing is usually offered at 24–28 weeks of pregnancy except when there is a history of previous gestational diabetes, when it should be offered at 18 weeks and, if negative, again at 26–28 weeks. The 75-g GTT is standard; the test should be done with the woman having fasted for the previous 8 hours. The fasting glucose level should be 5.5 mmol/L or less and 8.0 mmol/L or less 2 hours following the glucose load. Figures above these indicate a diagnosis of GDM.

What will be included in your initial discussion with Dora?

You need to assess Dora's general health and the progress of her pregnancy so far. Dora reports that she is well and feeling fetal movements but she wants to know what her test results mean. You explain that high sugar levels in the blood can bring about accelerated growth of the baby and cause problems following birth. It is important that her blood sugar levels are well controlled for the rest of her pregnancy. Dora will attend the combined antenatal–diabetic clinic and be under the care of the diabetic pregnancy team of your maternity unit. Dora has a good understanding of diabetes—she tells you that her mother has diabetes and she herself understands how to use a glucometer.

What examination does Dora need at this visit?

You carry out a routine antenatal check for Dora. Her blood pressure is normal; the uterine fundal height is 30 cm, a little large for dates. Dora has had an 18-week ultrasound scan that confirmed her dates and showed no fetal abnormality; the placenta was noted to be fundal. You order a further scan to assess fetal growth. The diabetes educator spends some time with Dora discussing diet and explaining the use of the glucometer. Dora will keep a record of blood glucose levels before breakfast and at 2 hours following each meal over the next 2 weeks, and return for a further visit. She understands that it is desirable that BSLs are in the range 4–5.5 mmol/L fasting, <8.0 mmol/L at 1 hour and <7 mmol/L at 2 hours postprandially (Fig. 27.1).

What are your concerns at following visits?

Two weeks later you see Dora again in the clinic. She continues to feel well—in fact, since sticking to a diet with less carbohydrate and fat she feels better than earlier in the pregnancy. Perusal of the blood sugar book shows pre-breakfast glucose levels of less than 5.5 mmol/L and all postprandial levels have been below 7.8 mmol/L. You congratulate Dora on her success in managing her condition. The ultrasound scan report shows the baby to be close to the 97th percentile when plotted on a fetal growth chart (Fig. 27.2). On physical examination the fundal height now measures 33 cm but is otherwise unremarkable.

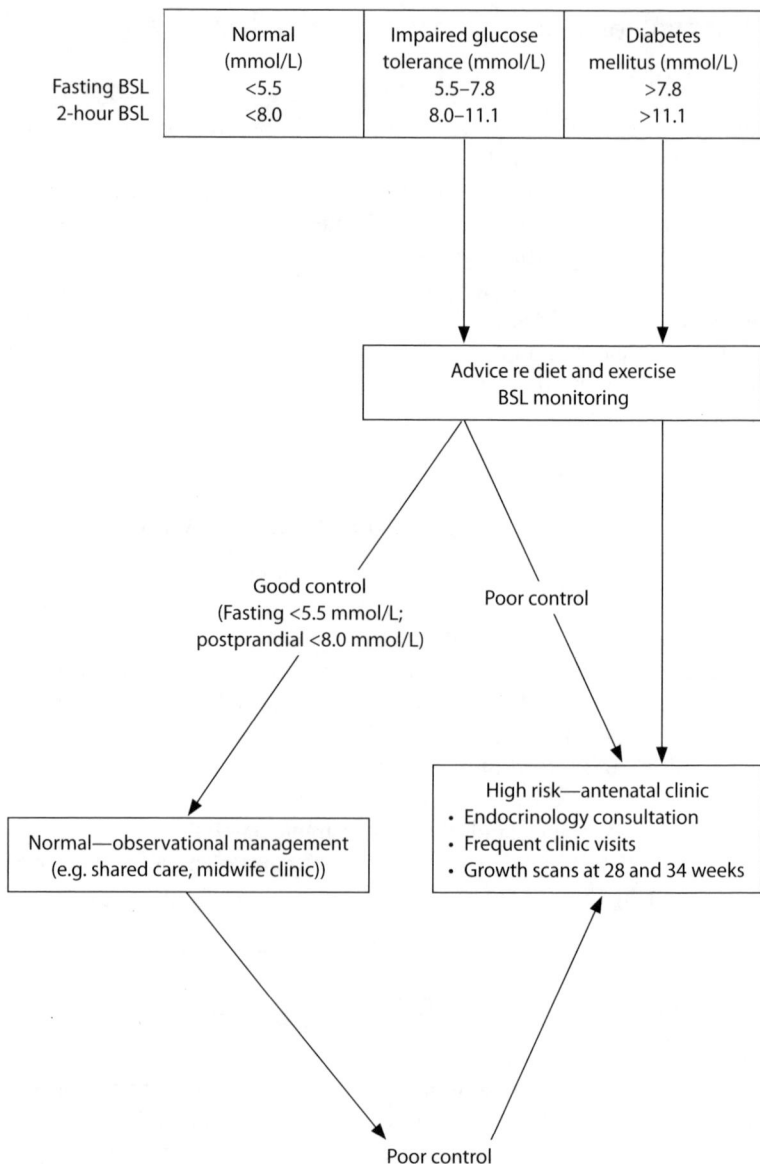

Figure 27.1 Flow chart for the management of abnormal glucose tolerance in pregnancy—75-g glucose tolerance test

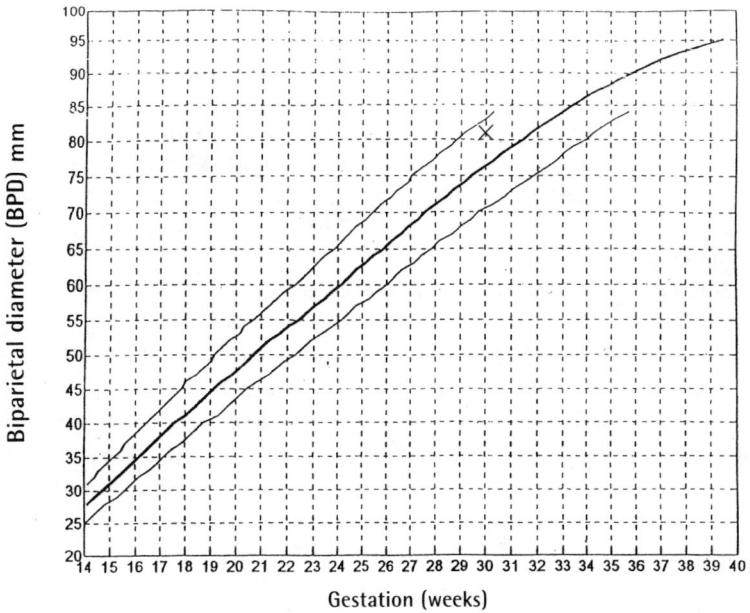

Figure 27.2 Fetal growth chart shows growth rates on the 50th percentile and 3rd and 97th percentiles on either side. The x indicates measurement of BPD at 30 weeks' gestation

Over the next 6 weeks Dora's glucose levels continue to be well controlled, fetal movements are normal and the baby continues to grow on clinical examination. A further ultrasound scan for growth assessment shows the growth progressing along the 90th percentile; Doppler scans and measurements of liquor volume are within normal limits.

At 36 weeks Dora returns to the clinic in some consternation—she tells you that despite sticking to her diet her blood sugar levels are rising—her fasting level is about 6 mmol/L and postprandial it is varying at about 8–11 mmol/L. After consultation with the endocrinologist attached to your clinic it is decided to commence Dora on insulin, starting with 16 units daily in divided doses. Instructions are given to Dora about insulin administration. Arrangements are made to see her in the day pregnancy unit to monitor her blood glucose level and adjust the insulin dosage as required, and for second-daily CTG monitoring.

Over the next 2 weeks Dora's insulin requirements increase substantially—to over 100 units daily. CTG monitoring continues to show a reactive trace and fetal movements are normal. However, at 38 weeks the fundal height measures 43 cm. A further ultrasound scan gives an estimated fetal weight (EFW) of 4400 g. On clinical examination the baby is noted to be a cephalic presentation but the head is high, five-fifths above the pelvic brim and very mobile. Dora herself is very concerned about the size of her baby, which she feels is greater than that of her first child, and about her ability to have a vaginal birth. You explain to Dora that given the fact that her diabetes is becoming difficult to control and the baby is larger than her first, with no possibility at present for induction of labour, you recommend an elective caesarean section, with close monitoring of the fetus until then. After some discussion about the details and risks of caesarean section Dora assures you she is happy with this plan.

What arrangements do you make for this procedure?

You arrange admission for the following day—Dora will fast from midnight, omit her normal morning dose of insulin and come into the birth suite at 7 am. The operation is scheduled for 9 am. You order an FBC and group and hold for Dora. Anaesthesia is discussed with her—she requests regional anaesthesia and will bring her partner Francisco as her support person in the operating theatre. You explain to Dora what will happen during the surgery, the risks of caesarean section, and what she can expect to feel after the operation—she will have an epidural cannula inserted for the anaesthetic, which can be left in postoperatively for analgesia, which she herself can control.

Risks of caesarean section

- Anaesthetic risks—anaesthesia is more commonly regional but women must be aware of the possibility that general anaesthesia may be required
- Haemorrhage—consent should be obtained from all women for blood transfusion or if this is declined this should be discussed and noted
- Infection—of operation site, urinary tract infection, pulmonary infection related to anaesthesia, distant infection
- Damage to adjacent organs, in particular bladder and bowel
- Thromboembolic complications
- Rarely, need for hysterectomy

The following morning Dora presents to the birth suite as planned. She feels well, the baby is moving normally and a short CTG strip shows a normal reactive pattern. An intravenous line is established and Dora is commenced on infusions of glucose and insulin, with hourly BSLs. The infusion rate is adjusted to keep the BSLs within the range 4–7 mmol/L. (Insulin infusions consist of soluble insulin 50 units [0.5 mL] made up to 50 mL with normal saline, and dextrose 5%, run via the same cannula with dextrose as the main infusion and insulin 'piggy-backed' as the secondary line. Other fluids should be administered through separate lines.) At 8.30 am Dora is transferred to the operating suite, where a combined epidural–spinal anaesthetic is put into place. A lower segment caesarean section is performed by your consultant, resulting in the birth of a baby boy weighing 4700 g. The baby is in good condition, with Apgar scores of 8 at 1 minute and 9 at 5 minutes and is handed to Dora; however, after some minutes he appears to have mild respiratory distress so is transferred to the special care nursery for observation. Over the next 3 days the baby remains in the nursery, being treated for mild respiratory distress and hypoglycaemic episodes, but by day 3 he is well enough to be transferred back to the postnatal ward with his mother. Breastfeeding is establishing well.

What care does Dora need postnatally?

Postnatally Dora continues on the insulin–glucose infusion until she is able to eat, which she is able to do 7 hours after the operation. BSLs are taken hourly and, in fact, her insulin requirements fall rapidly to zero. Otherwise her postnatal course is uneventful, the wound heals well, the subcuticular suture is removed on day 5 and Dora is able to go home with her baby, arrangements having been made for the community midwife to call daily over the following days.

Before discharge arrangements are made for Dora to attend her general practitioner at 6 weeks and to have further GTT. You explain to her that she is predisposed to develop type 2 diabetes in later life.

Clinical pearls

- Tight glucose control is the key to a successful outcome in pregnancy in diabetic women.

References and further reading

Creasy R, Resnik R, eds. Maternal–Fetal Medicine—Principles and Practice. 5th edn. Philadelphia: WB Saunders, 2004:1023–42, 1045–56.

Hoffman L, Nolan C, Wilson JD et al. Gestational diabetes mellitus—management guidelines (consensus statement). The Australasian Diabetes in Pregnancy Society. Med J Aust 1998; 169:93–7.

Scollan-Koliopoulos M, Guadagno S, Walker EA. Gestational diabetes management: guidelines to a healthy pregnancy. Nurse Pract 2006; 31(6):14–23.

Society of Obstetricians and Gynaecologists of Canada. Clinical Practice Guidelines: Screening for Gestational Diabetes. Available online at www.socg.org.

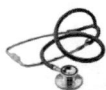

Case 28
Diane has diabetes and is pregnant …

In the combined antenatal–diabetic clinic you carry out a booking visit for Diane. Diane is a 27-year-old primigravida who has been a type 1 diabetic since the age of 11. She is now 8 weeks advanced in this pregnancy. Prior to her pregnancy she worked hard with her general practitioner to make sure that her blood sugar levels were tightly controlled, with fasting levels at 4–5.5 mmol/L and postprandial at or below 7.8 mmol/L. She also had baseline renal function tests, which are normal with no evidence of increased urinary protein excretion, and ophthalmological examination has shown no retinal damage. She has been taking folic acid daily for the past 5 months and has had an ultrasound scan 2 weeks ago which shows a 6-week fetus and a fetal heartbeat present, all consistent with her dates. Her glycohaemoglobin (HbA$_{1c}$) level is within the reference range.

What other concerns are there for Diane early in her pregnancy?

Diane wants to know about tests for Down syndrome and other fetal abnormalities that might be done in the first trimester. You explain to her that such tests are available—that originally they tended to be offered to women over the age of 35 because Down syndrome and other rarer chromosomal abnormalities are more common with increasing maternal age, but that since Down syndrome can occur at any maternal age and as the tests are non-invasive they are increasingly being offered to younger women.

What information do you give Diane about early antenatal screening?

You further explain that the tests available are screening tests—that is, they are designed to select women whose infants are at risk of Down syndrome but they are not diagnostic of the condition. If Diane has the tests she will be given a risk assessment—if she is considered high risk she will be offered a diagnostic test, which will give her an answer that is virtually 100% accurate to her question—does my baby have Down syndrome? If she is found to be low risk, that in itself is not a guarantee that the baby is unaffected by Down syndrome but it is unlikely.

The tests, you tell Diane, are in two parts. Firstly, an ultrasound scan is done at 11–13 weeks in which the thickness of the skin fold on the back of the baby's neck is measured. The scan must be performed by a suitably trained and accredited sonographer. This measurement is the fetal nuchal translucency (FNT). It has been shown that an increased FNT is associated with an increased risk of Down syndrome and of certain other chromosomal defects (trisomy 13 and 18) and congenital heart defects. Secondly, a blood test is performed to measure certain biochemical markers: the free β subunit of human chorionic gonadotrophin (HCG) and pregnancy-associated plasma protein (PAPP-A). The two types of test result are put together with the maternal age and the level of risk is assessed. Using the FNT alone 70–80% of fetuses with Down syndrome and associated abnormalities will be assigned to the high-risk group; adding the biochemical tests to the FNT result increases the proportion to 90%.

Desirable characteristics of a screening test

- Non-invasive or minimal side effects (FNT and biochemical screening carry no risk to the fetus)
- The condition should not be rare in the population studied
- A treatment or management option for the condition being screened for must exist (termination of pregnancy can be offered to women with fetuses found to have Down syndrome or similar chromosomal abnormalities)
- The test must be cheap—large numbers of people must be screened with relatively few positives
- High sensitivity
- High specificity

Diane elects to have the combined test done and the results show that she is at low risk. She has 1 in 1333 risk of having an affected child; her age-related risk alone is 1 in 650. Diane decides not to proceed to any diagnostic testing.

How do you follow Diane's subsequent progress?

Diane is seen regularly at the combined antenatal–diabetic clinic so that both the progress of the pregnancy and her diabetic control can be assessed concurrently. Clinically all goes well—her blood pressure remains within the normal range, as does clinical assessment of uterine size. At 18 weeks Diane is referred to a tertiary centre for a fetal morphology ultrasound scan (USS). Normal morphology is reported.

At 24, 28, 32 and 36 weeks' growth USS is performed for Diane in your hospital and measurements of fetal growth are plotted on a growth chart. This shows satisfactory growth, with all measurements lying between the 10th and 90th percentiles. From 28 weeks' gestation measurements are also made of the amniotic fluid index (AFI) and Doppler ultrasound studies of umbilical artery blood flow are carried out.

The AFI is calculated by adding together the maximum amniotic fluid depths in each of the four quadrants of the uterus, as seen on ultrasound; the normal range in the third trimester is 7–20 cm. Umbilical arterial blood flow is expressed as the ratio of velocity in systole to that in diastole (S/D ratio). An increasing S/D ratio is evidence of increasing placental resistance. As placental resistance increases, diastolic flow can decrease, cease and eventually be reversed—these changes are evidence of chronic fetal hypoxia and perinatal mortality and morbidity are increased in these circumstances.

How is Diane's diabetes managed?

Insulin requirements are managed by the endocrine team in conjunction with the diabetic pregnancy clinic. Diane's insulin requirements, as expected, rise during her pregnancy but BSLs remain within the desired range; HbA_{1c} levels are assessed regularly.

Will Diane be permitted to go past term?

It is safest to arrange delivery by term, and frequently by 38 weeks' gestation, in an insulin-dependent diabetic. Intrauterine fetal death due to variations in glucose levels is increasingly a possibility in the last weeks of pregnancy. Pre-eclampsia may be a complication of pregnancy in diabetic women.

At 39 weeks Diane develops some mild hypertension, headache and proteinuria and a decision is made to induce labour. Vaginal examination shows the cervix to be unfavourable for artificial rupture of the membranes (ARM) so prostaglandin gel is inserted to bring about cervical ripening.

The following day the cervix is suitable for ARM and oxytocin induction. A glucose–insulin infusion is commenced prior to the induction and BSLs are performed hourly during labour, adjustments to the infusion rate being made to keep the BSL within the range 4–7 mmol/L. After a 6-hour labour Diane proceeds to the spontaneous vaginal delivery of a baby girl weighing 3900 g.

Postnatally Diane is kept on the glucose–insulin infusion with hourly BSLs performed but her insulin requirements quickly drop back to pre-pregnancy levels, she is able to eat normally and the infusion is discontinued. The baby is observed in the special care nursery for the management of hypoglycaemia but is able to return to her mother by day 2.

Clinical pearls

- The causes of mortality and morbidity in the babies of diabetic mothers include respiratory distress syndrome, hypoglycaemia, hypocalcaemia, hypomagnesaemia, jaundice and macrosomia leading to traumatic delivery. Level 3 nursery facilities may be required for the infants of diabetic mothers, particularly when there has been poor glucose control or where delivery takes place before 36 weeks' gestation.

References and further reading

Jovanovic L, Nakai Y. Successful pregnancy in women with type 1 diabetes: from preconception through postpartum care. Endocrinol Metab Clin North Am 2006; 35(1):79–97, vi.

McElduff A, Cheung NW, McIntyre HD et al. The Australasian Diabetes in Pregnancy Society consensus guidelines for the management of type 1 and type 2 diabetes in relation to pregnancy. Med J Aust 2005; 183(7):373–7.

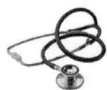

Case 29
Maria is followed through a twin pregnancy …

You are conducting an antenatal clinic when you first meet Maria, 38 years old and 14 weeks advanced in her fifth pregnancy. Maria has had a diagnosis of twin pregnancy made by her general practitioner at 8 weeks. She has had an ultrasound at 11 weeks, which has confirmed a continuing twin pregnancy. The pregnancy is dichorionic. Fetal nuchal translucency has been measured for each twin and is not abnormal for either. Her general practitioner has explained the possibility of chorionic villous sampling or amniocentesis for fetal chromosomal abnormality in view of Maria's age. After discussion with her husband Maria has decided not to have any further testing for fetal abnormality apart from the routine 18-week ultrasound scan.

What further information is related to your immediate care of Maria?

Maria has been experiencing marked nausea and vomiting but this now seems to be lessening. She has had four normal full-term pregnancies in the past and four spontaneous vaginal deliveries of healthy boys. There is no other relevant medical or family history. Maria is taking an iron–folate preparation. She is as yet unaware of fetal movements.

General examination is unremarkable, with a BP of 120/80 mmHg. The uterine fundus measures just to the level of the umbilicus and fetal heart tones are audible with Doppler scan, although you explain to Maria that you cannot with certainty identify two separate heartbeats. You order her 18-week ultrasound scan and arrange to see her following this.

What are the important points for following antenatal visits?

At 18 weeks Maria reports that she is well. She is feeling frequent fetal movements. Her ultrasound report confirms the dichorionic and hence diamniotic pregnancy; both fetuses are the expected size for 18 weeks and no abnormality has been demonstrated. The placentas appear fused, they lie posteriorly and fundal, well away from the lower pole of the uterus.

You arrange for Maria to have further ultrasound scans for fetal growth at 28, 32 and 36 weeks. You explain that intrauterine growth retardation is not uncommon with one or both twins, although it is more likely with mono-chorionic twins. In such cases and particularly with the rare monoamniotic twin pregnancy, twin-to-twin transfusion syndrome may occur because of vascular anastomoses within the two placentas.

How do you monitor progress of the pregnancy?

Maria is seen regularly from 24 to 36 weeks, and all observations are within normal limits. No vaginal bleeding or excessive discharge is reported and her blood pressure is always within the normal range. The growth scans at 24, 28, 32 and 36 weeks are performed as planned. All show growth of both babies within the 10th and 90th percentiles. At 36 weeks both babies are presenting cephalically.

Possible complications of late pregnancy with twins include pre-eclampsia, gestational diabetes, antepartum haemorrhage, retarded intrauterine growth and the onset of preterm labour.

How and when is delivery planned for Maria?

At 36 weeks you discuss with Maria probable arrangements for delivery. She is feeling extremely tired and uncomfortable. You agree that it may be reasonable to carry out induction of labour for her at 38–39 weeks. Insertion of an epidural cannula in early established labour is recommended because, although both babies are cephalic, there is sometimes the need for urgent operative delivery of the second twin.

The following Sunday evening you are called urgently to the birth suite. Maria has been admitted in spontaneous labour. Her husband Renato is with her. She reports that her membranes ruptured during family dinner. She has come straight in to the hospital—in the car contractions have become strong and regular and now she has an urge to push. The midwife in attendance, Doreen, has performed a vaginal examination and reports that the cervix is 9 cm dilated with the head of the first baby below the iliac spines. All Maria's observations, including blood pressure, pulse and temperature are normal; external fetal cardiac monitoring is in place and both fetal heart traces are reactive. You send for anaesthetic, paediatric and further obstetric assistance; however, almost immediately with a strong contraction the head of the first twin crowns and you rapidly conduct a normal delivery of a baby boy in excellent condition.

Palpation of the abdomen now shows the second twin to be lying longitudinally with the head presenting. Over the next 10 minutes there are two short, quite feeble contractions so you add oxytocin 5 units to the intravenous Hartmann's solution already in place. The fetal heart trace for the second twin is satisfactory. On vaginal examination at 12 minutes after delivery of the first twin you find the fetal head well applied to the cervix and at the level of the iliac spines. You rupture the membranes, the liquor is clear and 2 minutes later the second twin is born—a girl!

Knowing that Maria is at moderate-to-high risk of a postpartum haemorrhage (i.e. high parity, twin pregnancy) you order one ampoule of oxytocin/ergometrine IM and add a further 30 units of oxytocin to the intravenous infusion. The placentas are delivered and the uterus is felt to be well contracted.

Mode of birth in twin delivery

- If the first twin is a cephalic presentation, vaginal birth is possible. If the first twin is a malpresentation, elective caesarean section is advised.
- Risk during birth mainly relates to the second twin, and the interval until delivery of this twin following the first delivery.
- An experienced obstetrician should be present for all twin births.
- Paediatric and anaesthetic staff should also be present.
- Continuous electronic fetal heart rate monitoring of both twins is required.
- Elective epidural anaesthesia is strongly advised—if internal podalic version and breech extraction of the second twin is performed, anaesthesia is mandatory.
- There is an increased risk of primary postpartum haemorrhage due to uterine atony.

Clinical pearls

- All the minor discomforts of pregnancy and most complications of later pregnancy are more frequent in multiple pregnancy.

- Perinatal mortality is increased by a factor of six in twin pregnancy compared to singleton pregnancies; perinatal morbidities show similar increases.

References and further reading

Dodd J, Crowther C. Should we deliver twins electively at 37 weeks gestation? Curr Opin Obstet Gynecol 2005; 17(6):579–83.

Society of Obstetricians and Gynaecologists of Canada. Clinical Practice Guidelines: Management of Twin Pregnancies Parts 1 and 2. Available online at www.socg.org.

Taylor MJ. The management of multiple pregnancy. Early Hum Dev 2006; 82(6):365–70.

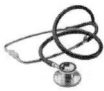

Case 30
Tayla presents with herpes in pregnancy ...

Tayla is a 17-year-old primigravida you are called to see in the birth suite late one Saturday night. Tayla is 33 weeks pregnant by a late ultrasound, being unsure of the date of her last menstrual period (LMP). She has booked at the antenatal clinic at about 25 weeks of pregnancy and made one subsequent visit to a general practitioner but otherwise has had no antenatal care. Tayla is accompanied by her mother but not by the father of her child, with whom she says she no longer has contact.

What history do you take from Tayla?

Tayla gives a history of a sudden gush of fluid from her vagina about an hour previously. She has also been experiencing burning and tingling in the perineum and now thinks she may have some sores in the area. From her notes you see that Tayla's routine blood and urine tests done at her booking visit were all unremarkable apart from a positive urine PCR test for chlamydia—Tayla has been prescribed azithromycin for this. Tayla is allergic to penicillin. She smokes more than 20 cigarettes a day.

What examination do you undertake?

You initially make a general examination of Tayla. Her blood pressure is 110/75 mmHg, pulse 70 bpm and temperature 37.6°C. Tayla appears mildly distressed and she complains of some period-like cramps as well as the perineal pain. Examination of her abdomen shows a uterine fundus 33 cm in height with a cephalic presentation, the uterus is soft and not tender and the fetal heart trace is reassuring. Palpation over the renal angles reveals some tenderness on the right.

Inspection of the vulva shows copious clear fluid consistent with amniotic fluid draining from the vagina. The posterior aspect of the left labium is inflamed and several vesicular lesions are present, two or three of which are blistered and weeping. The lesions extend onto the perineum as far as the anal margin. The appearance is typical of herpes genitalis (HSV-2) infection.

What are your concerns and how are these managed?

You explain the probable diagnosis to Tayla. 'Have you had previous episodes of herpes?', you ask. She denies this firmly. She is well aware of what herpes is. 'Will it affect my baby?', she asks. You answer that primary infections in the mother carry a high risk of infection of the baby if a vaginal birth occurs—50% develop encephalitis or generalised infection with major organ involvement and death. You ask about prodromal symptoms and Tayla admits to feeling some burning and tingling in the perineum for several days, but she had simply related this to the pregnancy. She is anxious about her baby's wellbeing, and asks if a caesarean section will be safer for the baby. You answer that this is indeed the case. While you have been talking with Tayla she has had two quite strong uterine contractions that were moderately painful and with each there has been a further gush of fluid from the vagina.

How do you proceed to a definite diagnosis of HSV-2?

You take swabs from two of the vesicular lesions after pricking each with a sterile needle. You explain to Tayla that it will be some time until you can get the results of these to confirm the diagnosis of herpes but that on the basis of the appearance of the lesions and the fact that she is becoming established in labour you recommend caesarean section as soon as it can be arranged. You will also commence her on a course of aciclovir and the baby will be given aciclovir after birth. You assure her that with caesarean delivery the baby's outlook is excellent.

> Preterm labour and birth (before 36 completed weeks of pregnancy) is associated with teenage pregnancy, underweight mothers, cigarette smoking, little antenatal care and maternal infection, including urinary tract infection (UTI) and bacterial vaginosis.

What other clinical problems does Tayla appear to have?

You also explain that she has signs of a UTI involving especially her right kidney, and that this may be what has precipitated early labour. A short general physical examination shows that her throat and lungs are clear, there is no mastitis or generalised lymphadenopathy and no tenderness or swelling of her calves. You obtain a midstream urine (MSU) specimen and after establishing an intravenous line prescribe cephalothin IV 6 hourly, observing her closely following the first dose to make sure there is no allergy to cephalosporin. You then make arrangements for an emergency caesarean section, obtaining consent, contacting the duty anaesthetist and paediatrician, taking blood for an FBC and group and hold, and inserting a urinary catheter. Tayla's mother will accompany her to the operating theatre.

Clinical comment

Urinary tract infection in pregnancy

- Common causes—urinary stasis and vesico–ureteric reflux associated with progesterone and other pregnancy hormones, and short female urethral length, predispose to infection by faecal organisms in particular.
- Asymptomatic infection, usually in the bladder, may become symptomatic and may ascend to involve the kidneys.
- UTI is a major predisposing cause of preterm labour.
- Recurrent infections may need prophylaxis for the remainder of the pregnancy; full urinary tract investigation postpartum is recommended.

A routine caesarean section is performed without incident and a baby girl delivered, weight 2200 g, Apgar scores of 7 at 1 minute and 10 at 5 minutes. The baby is transferred to the special care baby nursery for observation.

> The principal risks to the baby from preterm birth are respiratory distress syndrome due to relative deficiency of surfactant; intraventricular haemorrhage; hyperbilirubinaemia and jaundice with the risk of kernicterus; infection owing to the poorly developed immune system; and hypoglycaemia as the preterm infant has relatively low glycogen stores.

What is your ongoing plan for Tayla and her baby?

The baby progresses well over the ensuing few days, there is no evidence of neonatal herpes and breastfeeding is established. Results of the investigations you ordered antenatally are now received—PCR testing on swabs from the vulval lesions is positive for HSV-2, and the MSU shows growth of *Escherichia coli* sensitive to cephalosporins. In view of her age and single status you arrange for Tayla to be seen by the hospital's adolescent team social worker and appropriate support to be provided on discharge. You also refer Tayla to the sexual health clinic for follow-up and management should she experience recurrent episodes of genital herpes and for possible contact tracing. You discuss various appropriate methods of contraception with Tayla. She wishes to breastfeed her daughter for several months so you suggest either the progestogen rod implant or medroxyprogesterone, but you emphasise also the importance of using condoms to reduce the chances of contracting further sexually transmitted infections (STIs) if she is not in a mutually monogamous relationship. You also discuss ways of reducing cigarette consumption, which Tayla has indicated she wishes to do. You stress how important it is for her infant daughter to avoid passive smoking and explain that the baby was smaller than expected possibly because of Tayla's cigarette smoking during pregnancy. Tayla seems keen to follow your advice.

Clinical comment

Acquisition of HSV-2 in pregnancy occurs in 0.3–3% of women depending on the population surveyed. Primary infection in the first half of pregnancy may cause a spontaneous abortion. Primary infection later in pregnancy may be associated with intrauterine growth retardation and/or preterm labour. Primary infections in pregnancy may be safely treated with aciclovir. Neonatal herpes occurs as a direct result of contact of the baby with maternal lesions during delivery; the risk is highest from primary infections. It is probable that maternal antibodies cross the placenta and protect the fetus so that in subsequent infections the risk of fetal infection is greatly reduced (from 50% to 3–5% of cases). Caesarean section is therefore recommended only for primary infection and in subsequent infections where extensive vulval/perineal involvement makes protecting the infant from lesions difficult. Caesarean section should be performed within 4 hours of rupture of the membranes. In women with recurrent herpes infections prophylaxis using aciclovir or valaciclovir from 36 weeks has been shown significantly to reduce the incidence of recurrent infection.

Clinical pearls

- Preterm birth occurs in 5–10% of all pregnancies and this figure has changed little in the past 20 years despite the more frequent use of tocolytics. Previous preterm birth is a positive predictor of a similar problem in a future pregnancy; education about quitting cigarette smoking, promoting a healthy lifestyle and prompt treatment of any infections during pregnancy may contribute to prevention.

References and further reading

Arbuckle TE, Sherman GJ. Comparison of the risk factors for pre-term delivery and intrauterine growth retardation. Paediatr Perinat Epidemiol 1989; 3(2):115–29.

Czaja CA, Hooton TM. Update on acute uncomplicated urinary tract infection in women. Postgrad Med 2006; 119(1):39–45.

Jungmann E. Genital herpes. Clin Evid 2005; 14:1937–49.

Khandelwal M. Genital herpes complicating pregnancy. Obstet Gynecol 2006; 107(3):740–1.

Roberts D, Dalziel S. Antenatal corticosteroids for accelerating fetal lung maturation for women at risk of preterm birth. Cochrane Database Syst Rev 2006; 3:CD004454.pub2.

Royal College of Obstetricians and Gynaecologists. Clinical Green-top Guidelines: Genital Herpes in Pregnancy—Management. Available online at www.rcog.org.uk.

Sheffield JS, Hill JB, Hollier LM et al. Valacyclovir prophylaxis to prevent recurrent herpes at delivery: a randomized clinical trial. Obstet Gynecol 2006; 108(1):141–7.

Sheffield JS, Hollier LM, Hill JB et al. Acyclovir prophylaxis to prevent herpes simplex virus recurrence at delivery: a systematic review. Obstet Gynecol 2003; 102(6):1396–403.

Vazquez JC, Villar J. Treatments for symptomatic urinary tract infections during pregnancy. Cochrane Database Syst Rev 2006; 3:CD002256.

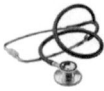

Case 31
Amanda suffers a placental abruption …

Amanda is a 32-year-old woman you are called to see in the birth suite. Amanda is at term in her second pregnancy and has brought herself to birth suite with a history of mild contractions every 3–4 minutes over the past 3 hours. Amanda is keen to have a water birth and after admission and checking of her vital signs by a midwife she has entered the spa bath where she is being supported by her partner, mother and 5-year-old daughter. She has, however, now developed some constant upper abdominal pain.

What is your initial management?

To conduct an adequate examination you must ask Amanda to get out of the bath and into a hospital bed. You take a short but pertinent history, having scrutinised the antenatal notes, and determined that the pregnancy has progressed normally and that her previous delivery was a spontaneous vaginal birth at 40 weeks' gestation following a labour of 5 hours.

Fetal movements have been normal. Amanda reports the sudden onset of dull pain over the upper part of the uterus. The pain is continuous and is unlike the mild pain of contractions which she is now experiencing more strongly. There is no associated nausea or vomiting.

Amanda's blood pressure is 120/80 mmHg, unchanged from her admission, and her pulse rate is 92 bpm. Palpation of the abdomen reveals tenderness and hardness over the fundus of the uterus. The lower part of the uterus is soft and non-tender and you are able to palpate the fetal head, of which three-fifths is above the pelvic brim.

What is your next step?

You need to check immediately on fetal wellbeing. A CTG is performed, which shows a baseline fetal heart rate of 175 bpm with good variability, acceleration with contractions and no decelerations.

What is your clinical impression?

It is likely that there has been a degree of placental abruption with some separation of the placenta from the uterine wall. This has led to fetal tachycardia and there exists the possibility that the abruption may extend, with further fetal compromise and even acute fetal distress.

How can this diagnosis be confirmed and what further steps are indicated?

You confirm your clinical diagnosis with a portable ultrasound scan, which shows some separation of the placenta and a small retroplacental clot. You also establish intravenous access and take blood for an FBC and coagulation screen.

> In placental abruption of moderate-to-severe degree a coagulation screen should be performed.

Do you perform a vaginal examination?

Yes—you need to know whether Amanda is established in labour and, if so, how far she has progressed. You explain to her your clinical impression and the fact that because the abruption may extend you wish to expedite delivery. You perform the vaginal examination and find that the cervix is 4 cm dilated, fully effaced and well applied to the fetal head. To accelerate labour and to check the colour of the liquor you rupture the membranes—some fresh meconium and some bright blood are expelled. You apply a scalp electrode and continue CTG monitoring—the fetal heart rate settles to 155 bpm with good variability and no decelerations.

> Women presenting with clinical signs of placental abruption and no evidence of fetal distress may be permitted to attempt vaginal delivery under close surveillance. If there is definite fetal distress and the woman is not close to full dilatation, then caesarean section may be the most appropriate action.

How do you continue to monitor the labour?

You explain to Amanda and her family the need for continuous monitoring—she has moved from a low-risk situation to a high-risk one. If the CTG trace becomes abnormal, then fetal scalp blood pH and lactate levels can be performed to assess the baby's wellbeing. Within 10 minutes of ARM Amanda is having stronger and more regular contractions and she begins to use nitrous oxide inhalation for pain relief. Monitoring continues for another hour with no significant abnormalities detected. At this point Amanda is feeling an urge to push.

Should Amanda have a further vaginal examination?

Yes—if she has reached full dilatation, then delivery of the baby in good time with maternal effort is desirable. If the cervix is not fully dilated Amanda should be discouraged from pushing.

Vaginal examination shows the cervix to be fully dilated with the head 1 cm below the ischial spines in the left occipito-anterior position. At this point the fetal heart rate tracing begins to show some prolonged decelerations down to 100 bpm with and following contractions, returning only briefly to the baseline of 160 bpm.

What are the implications of this change and what action should be taken?

These are 'type 2 dips'—prolonged decelerations to below a normal baseline rate indicating fetal hypoxia and the need to deliver the baby immediately.

Immediate delivery can be achieved by vacuum extraction (Fig. 31.1). After briefly explaining the need for urgent delivery to Amanda and calling a neonatal paediatrician, the bladder is emptied with a catheter. Amanda uses nitrous oxide inhalation during the catheterisation and with the application of the vacuum cup. This is applied over the flexion point of the baby's scalp and the vacuum pump employed. With the next contraction maternal effort is encouraged and downward traction exerted via the vacuum handle. Rotation of the head to the occipito-anterior position and some descent occurs. With two further contractions the head crowns and the baby is born. The baby is handed to the paediatrician. The birth is followed by a gush of fresh blood and clots.

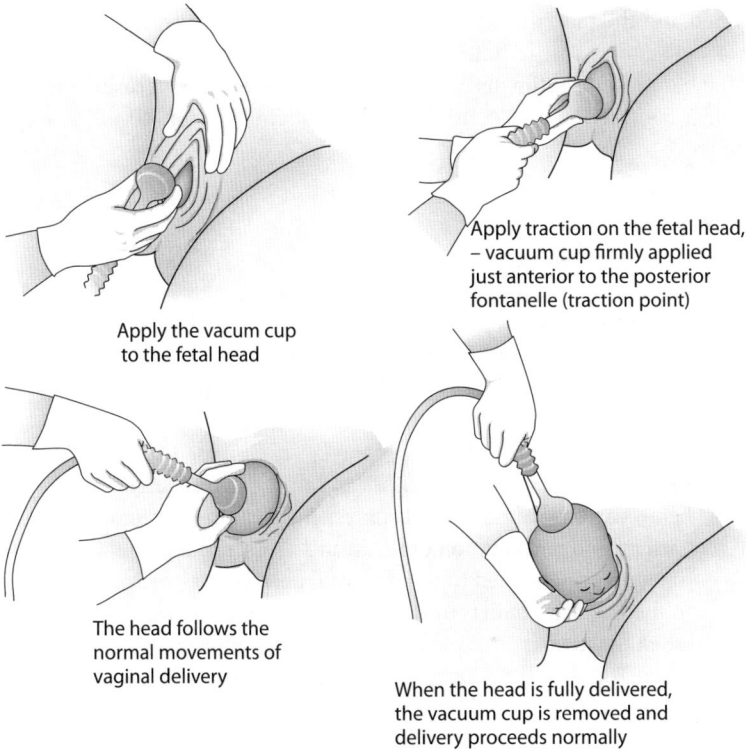

Apply the vacuum cup to the fetal head

Apply traction on the fetal head, – vacuum cup firmly applied just anterior to the posterior fontanelle (traction point)

The head follows the normal movements of vaginal delivery

When the head is fully delivered, the vacuum cup is removed and delivery proceeds normally

Figure 31.1 Use of the vacuum extractor in delivery

What is your immediate concern?

Amanda is at risk of a postpartum haemorrhage following an intrapartum haemorrhage. The abruption will have been associated with infiltration of blood among the myometrial fibres, which are thus less well able to contract down postpartum. With more major degrees of abruption, depletion of clotting factors may contribute to the development of postpartum haemorrhage.

How do you manage this situation?

Active management of the third stage of labour is essential. You give one ampoule of Syntometrine IM and add 40 units of oxytocin to 1 L of Hartmann's solution to be given intravenously. Signs of placental separation are noted and the placenta is delivered by controlled cord traction. With the placenta comes a large clot of dark blood, confirming your diagnosis. The total blood loss is estimated at 800 mL. You massage the uterus to establish a firm contraction and continue with oxytocin infusion 40 units over 8 hours.

Clinical pearls

- Postpartum haemorrhage continues to be a major cause of maternal mortality and morbidity in both developed and developing countries. Anticipation and active prophylaxis combined with aggressive management of active haemorrhage is the key to reducing the incidence of this common problem.
- Either the vacuum extractor or forceps can be used to effect delivery rapidly when fetal distress arises and the head has descended to below the level of the ischial spines. The vacuum extractor assists with flexion and rotation of the head so that a smaller fetal head diameter is presented to the maternal pelvic outlet. Forceps add to the expulsive efforts of the mother. Forceps can only be used when the head is in or close to the occipito-anterior (OA) position, whereas the vacuum extractor, because it assists with rotation, can be used with the head in positions other than OA.

References and further reading

Cotter A, Ness A, Tolosa J. Prophylactic oxytocin for the third stage of labour. Cochrane Database Syst Rev 2006; 3.CD001808.

Lurie S, Glezerman M, Bader C et al. Decision-to-delivery interval for instrumental vaginal deliveries: vacuum extraction versus forceps. Arch Gynecol Obstet 2006; 274(1):34–6.

Royal College of Obstetricians and Gynaecologists. Clinical Green-top Guidelines: Operative Vaginal delivery. Available online at www.rcog.org.uk.

Tikkanen M, Nuutila M, Hiilesmaa V et al. Clinical presentation and risk factors of placental abruption. Acta Obstet Gynecol Scand 2006; 85(6):700–5.

Vacca A. Vacuum-assisted delivery. Best Pract Res Clin Obstet Gynaecol 2002; 16(1):17–30.

Vacca A. Vacuum-assisted delivery: an analysis of traction force and maternal and neonatal outcomes. Aust N Z J Obstet Gynaecol 2006; 46(2):124–7.

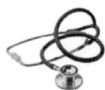

Case 32
Melissa has persistent vomiting in pregnancy ...

Melissa is a 22-year-old woman you are first called to see one Saturday afternoon in the emergency department. She has been referred by a local medical centre at 8 weeks of pregnancy because of persistent vomiting. The referring doctor also noted that Melissa appears very pale.

When you arrive in the emergency department you find Melissa leaning over a bowl, retching and spitting up bile-stained fluid. Her partner Nat and 1-year-old son are with her. You observe that she does, indeed, look pale and her skin is very dry.

Nat tells you that she has been vomiting increasingly frequently for the past 2 weeks. She has not eaten any solid food in this time. Initially she was able to tolerate fluids, mostly flat lemonade and water, but since yesterday he has not seen her drink anything. Over the past 2 weeks she has tried ginger tablets and antihistamines with no success. Nat also tells you that Melissa suffered nausea and vomiting during her last pregnancy but not to the current extent.

Nausea and/or vomiting are common symptoms of early pregnancy, particularly between 6 and 14 weeks. Although often referred to as 'morning sickness', symptoms may occur at any time and be provoked by various foods and other factors and relieved by a variety of measures. The condition is poorly understood; it has been attributed to the rapid rise in β-HCG and oestriol levels in early pregnancy, but psychological factors are probably also involved.

How do you proceed in this situation?

First you take a history from Melissa. She is sure of the date of her LMP. She was taking the COCP but missed 'a couple'. She had a pregnancy test performed at the medical centre 2 weeks ago and the result was positive. She was shocked to find that she was pregnant and is not sure how they will cope. They are currently living in a caravan park and Nat is unemployed.

Her son Josh was born by caesarean section for failure to progress in labour. He was not breastfed and she commenced on the COCP 6 weeks after his birth. She is not on any medications, has no other relevant medical history and no allergies. Melissa smokes 15 cigarettes a day.

What examination do you make of Melissa?

A good general examination is indicated. Melissa's conjunctivae, mucous membranes and nail beds are pale. Her BP is 90/60 mmHg and pulse is 100 bpm. She feels dizzy standing up. Her skin on closer inspection is very dry and her tongue dry and furred. Examination of the respiratory and cardiovascular systems and the abdomen is unremarkable.

What is the next step in your management of Melissa?

Melissa needs blood taken for FBC, urea and electrolytes and LFTs. She needs rehydration, which will need to be done intravenously. She needs anti-emetic therapy. You explain all this to Melissa and Nat, including the fact that Melissa requires admission to hospital. You also offer to arrange for a social worker to speak to the couple on the following Monday for assistance with their accommodation and financial problems.

Melissa is admitted to the ward and given Hartmann's solution 1 L 6-hourly for fluid replacement and metoclopramide 10 mg 6-hourly IM as required for vomiting. Initially she is given nothing by mouth.

What further investigations are indicated?

An MSU should be performed to exclude a UTI as a cause of vomiting. An ultrasound scan should be performed as soon as possible to rule out multiple pregnancy and trophoblastic disease as causes of hyperemesis.

Melissa's investigations show no evidence of a UTI. Electrolytes are within the normal range, as are LFTs. Ultrasound shows a single fetus with a CRL consistent with 8 weeks of pregnancy. The haemoglobin level is 90 g/L—despite the haemoconcentration associated with dehydration. A blood film shows hypochromic microcytic anaemia. Iron studies are ordered and low serum iron levels confirmed.

What is Melissa's subsequent progress?

As in most cases of hyperemesis Melissa settles quickly on this regimen. Within 12 hours she is tolerating oral fluids. You prescribe pyridoxine 50 mg twice daily for ongoing nausea.

Treatment of severe hyperemesis of pregnancy

- Parenteral promethazine or prochlorperazine may be used as alternatives to metoclopramide.
- Parenteral use of ondansetron may be considered in resistant cases. Ondansetron is a B3 category drug in pregnancy, which means that although no adverse effects are known in humans, it should only be used as second-line therapy.

What follow-up do you arrange for Melissa?

Melissa is discharged home well in 3 days' time with an appointment for follow-up in the antenatal clinic and arrangements for accommodation having been made by the social work department. She is tolerating an oral iron–folate preparation and has been advised to have frequent small meals of bland food. She has had a consultation with the hospital dietitian to discuss healthy eating habits for herself and her family.

Clinical pearls

- Psychological and environmental factors may contribute to the onset and severity of nausea and vomiting of pregnancy, and may require as much attention as clinical management of the condition.

References and further reading

Kirk E, Papageorghiou AT, Condous G, Bottomley C, Bourne T. Hyperemesis gravidarum: is an ultrasound scan necessary? Hum Reprod 2006; 21(9):2440–2.

Munch S, Schmitz M. Hyperemesis gravidarum and patient satisfaction: a path model of patients' perceptions of the patient–physician relationship. J Psychosom Obstet Gynaecol 2006; 27(1):49–57.

Society of Obstetricians and Gynaecologists of Canada. Clinical Practice Guidelines: The Management of Nausea and Vomiting of Pregnancy. Available online at www.socg.org.

Tan PC, Jacob R, Quek KF, Omar SZ. Indicators of prolonged hospital stay in hyperemesis gravidarum. Int J Gynaecol Obstet 2006; 93(3):246–7.

Case 33
Julia has a breech presentation …

Julia is a 32-year-old primigravida whom you meet for the first time in the antenatal clinic at 36 weeks' gestation. Julia has booked for a home delivery with an independent midwife, Thalia, who has been providing her antenatal care. Julia has made one visit to book in your hospital antenatal clinic—the hospital requires this visit if women are to be referred in later pregnancy or labour. That visit, at 7 weeks, revealed Julia to be a healthy woman with no relevant medical or surgical history. Julia runs her own media relations company and is extremely well informed about birthing options and patient rights.

What history do you take from Julia?

You need to establish why Julia has been referred to the antenatal clinic at this point in her pregnancy. At 34 weeks Thalia has queried whether the presentation is breech. Two days ago at Julia's 36-week visit she was still uncertain but yesterday afternoon an ultrasound scan confirmed that the baby is lying in the breech position with the legs fully extended along the body. The placenta is posterior, not low-lying. The estimated fetal weight (at 36 weeks) is 3900 g. Thalia has referred Julia to the hospital clinic and she has come along with her partner Damian, her mother and a friend, Kathleen.

How do you proceed with this consultation?

You check Julia's shared care card, which shows that there has been no abnormal bleeding during the pregnancy, her blood pressure has always been within normal limits and the fundal height has been increasing as expected. You ask about fetal movements—they are being felt as usual. You outline to Julia and Damian why Julia has been referred and she states that even if the baby remains in breech position she wants to try for a home birth.

You suggest to Julia that you re-check the baby's position and she agrees. Abdominal palpation reveals a very prominent head easily felt in the right upper quadrant but to be certain you use the portable ultrasound to demonstrate the breech presentation to all present.

You then explain to Julia and Damian the risks of breech presentation in labour; in particular, the fact that since moulding cannot occur there is no opportunity to test the size of the head against that of the mother's pelvis. If the head does not fit through safely, there is a 1 in 20 risk of neonatal death or brain damage associated with vaginal birth.

You should also explain that cord prolapse is more common with breech presentation.

Julia has been researching breech presentation on the Internet and points out that many breech babies have been successfully born vaginally. Julia's mother intervenes to say that her own sister had two breech deliveries quite safely; one of those children is now successful in insurance and the other is a wife and mother. Kathleen also has a friend who successfully birthed her third child as a breech.

What is your response to these comments?

You agree with all this but draw attention to the Term Breech Trial published in *The Lancet* in 2000, which demonstrated a three-fold increase in mortality and morbidity among breech babies of mothers assigned to attempt vaginal delivery compared to those delivered by planned caesarean section. You explain that while many, indeed most, breech babies can probably be safely born vaginally, a significant number will suffer death or damage and that we currently have no really accurate way of determining which these are. There is therefore a greater risk for Julia's baby if she attempts vaginal delivery with the baby in a breech presentation than there would be with a cephalic presentation. Furthermore, in a home delivery without ready access to experienced obstetric care the risks are much greater should a problem arise. Already the baby weighs close to 4000 g and by term could be expected to be well above 4000 g, which poses an additional risk. As this is Julia's first baby there is not the comfort of knowing as one might with a multipara that she has previously safely delivered an infant of weight greater than 4000 g as a cephalic presentation.

What other options are available to Julia?

You further explain that while elective caesarean section is a definite safe option, there is also the possibility of attempting external cephalic version (ECV). This could be done the following week after confirming that the baby is still breech and performing a CTG to check fetal wellbeing. You tell

Julia that there is approximately a 40% chance that her baby will be turned to a cephalic presentation and that there is a small risk of damage to baby, placenta or cord that may necessitate immediate caesarean section. You also tell her that there is a possibility that the baby will turn spontaneously to a cephalic presentation any time up until labour starts, although because this is her first baby and the baby lies with the legs splinted along the body (frank breech) this is less likely than with a baby with the legs flexed (complete breech) in a multiparous woman.

Details and risks of external cephalic version

- Should be performed at about 36–37 weeks—before this the baby may turn spontaneously; after this the chances of success are reduced
- Perform with facilities close by for emergency caesarean section if needed
- Contraindications are antepartum haemorrhage, hypertension in pregnancy, uterine scar and multiple pregnancy
- Monitor the fetus before and after procedure
- A tocolytic is usually given 30 minutes before attempting the procedure
- Risks include direct damage to the baby, cord entanglement, placental abruption
- The procedure involves gently dislodging the buttocks and/or legs and feet of the baby from the mother's pelvis and 'somersaulting' the baby into cephalic presentation
- Rhesus negative mothers should be given anti-D prophylaxis

Damian asks, *'Why is the baby a breech?'*

You explain that the reasons for breech presentation aren't always well understood—sometimes there can be an obstruction low in the pelvis, such as a placenta praevia or a cervical fibroid or ovarian cyst, although this is not the case for Julia; sometimes there can be minor variations in the shape of the uterus—again this is not obvious in Julia's case as there is no evidence of a uterine septum or separate horn. Some babies seem to prefer

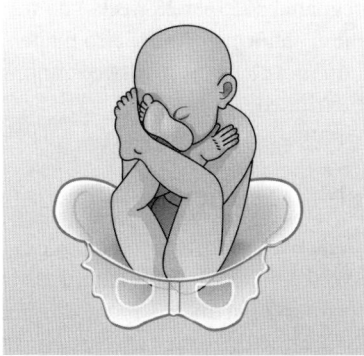

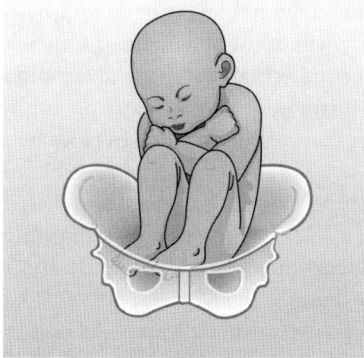

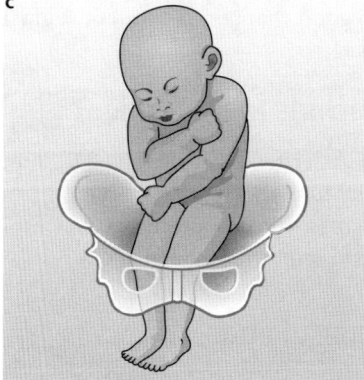

Figure 33.1 Types of breech presentation: **(a)** frank breech, **(b)** complete breech and **(c)** footling breech

this position and to remain in it to term, although many babies in breech position in earlier pregnancy (25% at 28 weeks) do turn spontaneously by 36–37 weeks. Congenital abnormalities are also higher in breech presentations, and as Julia chose not to have an 18-week anomaly ultrasound this possibility cannot be excluded.

Julia then asks about the details of caesarean section

You explain that an elective caesarean section would be done at about 39 weeks to try to avoid Julia going into labour early, thus avoiding an elective procedure becoming a semi-emergency, although you emphasise that this can be safely dealt with as the facilities for caesarean section are always available in the operating theatre. You outline the procedure for an elective caesarean—regional anaesthesia will be offered so Julia will be awake, the surgery will occur at a planned time with Damian present, she will be able to see the actual delivery and to hold and nurse her baby very soon after the birth. Only one support person will be allowed into the operating theatre but others can remain close by outside and see the baby as soon as feasible. It should also be possible for Julia to go home within 24 hours if mother and baby are well and there is adequate support at home. Thalia can also come into the operating theatre for the surgery and then be available for support postoperatively and at home postnatally. You explain that one lower segment caesarean section does not mean that future babies also need caesarean delivery—if a later child is in a cephalic presentation, then vaginal birth after caesarean section (VBAC) can safely be attempted with a good chance (60–70%) of vaginal delivery.

How do you conclude this interview?

You explain that you understand that attempted ECV and a possible caesarean section are very far from the couple's preferred option for the pregnancy. However, you ask them to think about what you have told them, which they are agreeable to, and to return the following day.

The following consultation

Julia now tells you that her main concern is the health of the baby. She and Damian consider the risks of ECV too high and she wishes to be booked for caesarean section, although if the baby turns spontaneously she will continue with her plans for a home birth.

What information must you give Julia about caesarean section?

Julia must be well informed about the risks of caesarean surgery. Having outlined these risks and given Julia an information leaflet about the surgery, you complete consent forms with her for the surgery in 2 weeks' time and arrange blood tests—FBC and group and hold—and an anaesthetic consultation. You assure Julia that the presentation of the baby will be assessed by ultrasound just prior to surgery to be certain that there has not been any last minute change. The couple are happy with this plan.

> The risks of caesarean section to the woman include anaesthetic risks—allergic/anaphylactic reactions to drugs, unsuccessful regional anaesthesia, aspiration, pneumonia—and the risks of the surgery itself—haemorrhage, infection, damage to adjacent organs and thromboembolism. There is a small risk that the woman may die (about 2 per 10 000 primary elective caesarean operations). There is also a small increase in the incidence of placenta praevia in subsequent pregnancies.

Two weeks later Julia presents for admission and you confirm the breech presentation and presence of the fetal heart. Julia is transferred to the operating theatre, where epidural anaesthesia is performed. You assist your consultant in an uneventful lower segment caesarean section, after which Julia returns to the maternity ward and the following day is discharged home to the care of her midwife.

One week later you are called to see Julia in the emergency department, where she has presented on the advice of her midwife. She complains of feeling feverish and generally unwell, and has pain in her left breast. On examination her temperature is 38°C, pulse 90 bpm and blood pressure 110/70 mmHg. Her chest is clear, the abdominal wound is clean and healing well, and there is no tenderness over the loins or calves. The right breast appears normal but the left is swollen and reddened, especially over the upper outer quadrant. It is hot and tender on palpation but there is no fluctuation; the overlying skin is shiny.

What is your clinical impression?

You make a diagnosis of mastitis and explain to Julia that although she can continue breastfeeding she should complete a full course of antibiotics to

195

prevent the infection developing into a breast abscess. Knowing that the most likely causative organism is *Staphylococcus aureus*, you prescribe a 10-day course of dicloxacillin, a paracetamol–codeine combination for pain relief and also suggest the use of warm packs. You arrange follow-up for Julia with both her midwife and her general practitioner.

Causes of postpartum pyrexia

- Urinary tract infection
- Endometritis
- Wound infection   at site of caesarean section, episiotomy or vaginal tear, cannula insertion for regional anaesthesia
- Basal atelectasis and pneumonia after anaesthesia for caesarean section
- Mastitis
- Deep venous thrombosis
- Incidental—influenza, chest infections, meningitis, endocarditis—always examine the whole woman!

Clinical pearls

- Breech babies may turn spontaneously to cephalic at any time up until the start of labour—always check the presentation immediately before performing a caesarean section when the indication is breech presentation.
- Women and their partners should be included as fully as possible in all decisions about pregnancy intervention—particularly elective caesarean section. Women's perceptions of involvement in decision making greatly influence their physical and emotional wellbeing postpartum.

References and further reading

Hannah ME, Hannah W, Hewson SA. Planned caesarean section versus planned vaginal birth for breech presentation at term: a randomised multicentre trial. Term Breech Trial Collaborative Group. Lancet 2000; 356(9239):1375–83.

Hofmeyr GJ, Gyte G. Interventions to help external cephalic version for breech presentation at term. Cochrane Database Syst Rev 2006; 3:CD000184.pub2.

Hofmeyr GJ, Hannah ME. Planned caesarean section for term breech delivery. Cochrane Database Syst Rev 2006; 3:CD000166.

Hutton EK, Hofmeyr GJ. External cephalic version for breech presentation before term. Cochrane Database Syst Rev 2006; 3:CD000084.pub2.

Royal College of Obstetricians and Gynaecologists. Clinical Green-top Guidelines: Breech Presentation—Management, and National Evidence-Based Guidelines: Caesarean Section. Both available online at www.rcog.org.uk.

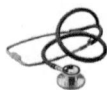

Case 34
Tegan develops an obstetric emergency ...

On a Sunday morning in birth suite, you are asked to see a 32-year-old woman, Tegan, who is 36 weeks' pregnant with her third child. Tegan has presented because she has had some irregular contractions overnight and is uncertain whether her waters have broken—she had a small gush of fluid vaginally earlier that morning. Her pregnancy to date has been unremarkable and the baby is moving normally but the midwife in attendance is concerned that the presentation is a breech.

How do you proceed with this consultation?

You review Tegan's antenatal notes and take a short but relevant history. In both previous pregnancies the babies were breech presentations up to 36–37 weeks but converted spontaneously to cephalic presentation. During this pregnancy the baby has been at times recorded as breech and at other times as cephalic. Tegan's blood pressure and other observations, including measurement of uterine fundus height, have been normal throughout the pregnancy. Results of all routine investigations have been normal apart from the fact that an MSU at booking showed a growth of group B *Streptococcus* (GBS). Tegan's blood group is O Rhesus negative and Tegan has been given anti-D 625 units at 28 and 34 weeks of pregnancy.

Tegan reports only slight vaginal loss since coming into the hospital and contractions have been infrequent (less than one in 10 minutes) and mild.

What examination do you conduct for Tegan?

All standard observations are normal. A short CTG trace has been performed by the midwife prior to your arrival and is variable and reactive. You proceed to abdominal examination. Inspection suggests a longitudinal lie, which is confirmed by palpation. You are confident that the fetal head can be felt in the upper right quadrant of the abdomen and that the presentation therefore is breech. The fetal buttocks can be palpated just above the pelvic brim. You use a portable ultrasound scanner to perform a scan, which confirms your diagnosis.

Should you perform a vaginal examination?

You must perform a vaginal speculum examination to try to ascertain whether the membranes have ruptured as this will determine whether your management is expectant or active. You perform the speculum examination under strict aseptic conditions with scrubbing and sterile gloving, and preparation of the perineum with an antiseptic wash. Your examination shows that the cervix appears partly effaced but closed. There is no pool of liquor visible in the posterior fornix after Tegan has been lying for some time on her back and no appearance of liquor via the cervix when you ask her to cough. You collect sterile swabs from the cervix for microscopy and culture.

What is your recommendation to Tegan?

You explain that you do not believe that she has ruptured the membranes nor is she in labour, but you wish to keep her for observation in case labour is, in fact, imminent. You explain to her the risks of breech presentation and give her some written information about this. She is already familiar with much of this from her previous pregnancies. You explain that she will be given penicillin prophylaxis to cover her delivery because of the finding of GBS earlier in the pregnancy. You arrange to transfer her to the antenatal ward for observation at least for some hours. She asks if her partner Peter can go home to arrange care for her other children and you assure them both that nothing is likely to happen in the next couple of hours. Peter can be contacted if the need arises. Tegan is duly transferred to the ward.

One hour later you are summoned urgently to the antenatal ward. Tegan has called the midwife because she has had a large gush of fluid vaginally and felt 'something coming down'. Immediate inspection by the midwife has shown a pulsating umbilical cord protruding from the vagina.

What do you do?

This is an acute obstetric emergency. Fetal death may result from compression of the cord between the presenting fetal part and the mother's pelvis or cervix. You urgently summon help from other midwifery staff, senior obstetric and anaesthetic personnel. You insert your gloved hand into the vagina to replace the cord and hold up the presenting part, the breech, as high as possible. You are assisted in this by midwifery staff, who turn Tegan into the knee–chest position. During these manoeuvres you explain to Tegan what is happening, assure her that you can feel the baby's heart beating through the cord pulsations and that the heart rate is normal. You further rapidly explain that as she is not in labour she will need an immediate caesarean section to deliver her baby and that this will need to be under general anaesthesia. With some difficulty you get a consent form signed—there is not time to give an adequate outline of the risks of the procedure.

At this point both your consultant and Tegan's family arrive. The consultant quickly explains the position to Peter. By then the anaesthetist has also arrived and asked for Tegan to be moved to the operating theatre. You accompany Tegan to theatre on the trolley with a hand still keeping the breech up away from the cord. You remain in this position until general anaesthesia has been induced and your consultant has performed a rapid abdominal and uterine incision and delivered a live female baby. Antibiotics are given routinely for caesarean section in your hospital in the form of cephalothin 2 g IV but in view of the high risk of infection in this case you add metronidazole 2 g.

The baby is in good condition and is handed to neonatal paediatric staff. The information is given to the paediatric staff that Tegan's earlier MSU showed GBS and that there was not time to administer penicillin intrapartum. It is decided that swabs will be taken from the baby, who will also be observed in the special care baby unit (SCBU). The operation proceeds uneventfully thereafter; however, you note that due to the urgent nature of the proceedings the use of calf compressors, normally routine for caesarean surgery, has been omitted. You include this in your writing up of the case and recommend early mobilisation and adequate fluid intake postpartum.

GBS infection is a significant cause of neonatal mortality and morbidity. Controversy, as yet unresolved by clinical trials, surrounds the issues of whether, when and how to screen and treat the whole pregnant population for the infection. Antepartum maternal colonisation with GBS is a recognised risk factor but antepartum antibiotics do not eliminate this risk. Rapid intrapartum diagnosis of GBS is unreliable; however, intrapartum antibiotics significantly reduce the risk of vertical transmission.

Management of GBS carriers in pregnancy

- All women known to be carriers of GBS or to have had a child affected by early-onset GBS disease should be treated with IV penicillin during labour, until delivery.
- In cases of penicillin allergy, clindamycin or erythromycin may be given.
- Antibiotics should also be given in labour to women with prolonged rupture of the membranes (>18 hours) or preterm labour at less than 35 weeks, and where the maternal temperature is 38°C or more.

What is your postoperative management of this case?

Later that day you visit Tegan. She is awake but she and her partner are still obviously quite shocked by the suddenness of the day's events. Peter is concerned that he was not permitted to be present at the birth and that he had not been contacted by the hospital when Tegan's membranes ruptured. Baby Plum is in the SCBU. Her blood has been tested and she has been found to be Rhesus positive, so anti-D 625 units have been administered to Tegan.

How do you deal with this couple's concerns?

You take some time to 'debrief' Tegan and Peter. You explain that cord prolapse is a recognised but unusual event occurring in about 1 in 800 births. There was no evidence of ruptured membranes or fetal distress when Tegan was examined in the birth suite but with the history she gave and with a breech presentation, observation close to specialist care was appropriate. You go over the events of the morning, explaining why it was necessary to perform an urgent caesarean section under general anaesthesia. Had the cord prolapse occurred at full dilatation with a cephalic presentation, operative vaginal delivery might have been possible, but even in that situation caesarean section under general anaesthesia may have been the safest and quickest option. You further explain that because Plum was born at 36 weeks' gestation she is experiencing some mild respiratory distress but that this is responding to simple measures in the SCBU and that you expect that the baby will be with her mother the following morning. You emphasise the urgency of the events to the couple and the fact that they have a live and healthy baby.

> After any unexpected or adverse event it is good practice to spend time 'debriefing' patients and their families. Not only does this provide relevant information to those concerned, it can also be beneficial to the doctor, particularly when there has been a neonatal or maternal death or serious morbidity. Good communication at the time of or soon after an event can help avoid subsequent litigation.

What further follow-up do you expect for Tegan?

Five days later you see Tegan again on your postnatal round. She appears well and happy and baby Plum is now with her. Breastfeeding is well established and it is expected that mother and baby will go home the following day. The abdominal wound is healing well and the subcuticular suture has been removed. However, Tegan is slightly febrile with a temperature of 37.8°C. Her temperature prior to this has been normal.

Is this significant?

You should take a short but relevant history and conduct an examination to ensure that there is no serious incipient cause for this temperature rise. There is no headache, cough or chest pain. On auscultation the chest is clear. There is no pain in the breasts, which are soft with no inflamed areas. There are no urinary or bowel symptoms. Tegan reports some abdominal tenderness around the wound site only and palpation shows an involuting uterus, which is only slightly tender, compatible with her recent surgery. There is no tenderness over the renal angles.

You then examine Tegan's legs. She states that there is some slight tenderness in her left calf but she did not think that this was important. On examination you find the calf is swollen and warm with tenderness on deep palpation.

> Postoperative pyrexia must always be taken seriously and a cause searched for. Where a laparotomy has been performed under general anaesthesia there is the possibility of respiratory and intra-abdominal complications, as well as urinary tract infection and thromboembolism, all directly related to the surgery. The possibility of incidental infection should also not be overlooked.

What are your concerns from this examination?

Symptoms and signs suggest the possibility of deep venous thrombosis (DVT) in the calf, possibly extending above the knee. If this is the case there is a risk of pulmonary embolism.

What is your immediate management?

You arrange a compression ultrasound for Tegan, which confirms DVT confined to the left calf.

Clinical comment

Acute venous thromboembolism (VTE) is a major cause of maternal mortality. The treatment of VTE in pregnancy has evolved rapidly over the past decade, with the introduction of new antithrombotic agents and growing experience and evidence for their use in pregnancy. This process is ongoing and it is desirable to involve the haematologist in the care of pregnant or recently pregnant women with VTE. In pregnancy, 85% of DVTs are left-sided compared to 55% in the non-pregnant.

What investigations should be performed?

A full thrombophilia screen should be performed for Tegan—testing for activated protein C resistance (APCR)/factor V (Leiden) gene mutation (FVL), protein C, protein S, antithrombin-3, elevated fasting homocysteine level, elevated factor VIII level, methyltetrahydrofolate reductase (MTHFR), factor II mutation, lupus anticoagulant and increased anticardiolipin antibodies. Most of these tests can be done before Tegan is commenced on anticoagulants but protein S and factor VIII cannot be measured in the acute phase of VTE and later repeat screening (after about 12 weeks) should be arranged, usually in conjunction with the haematologist.

What is your further management?

In consultation with the haematologist anticoagulation is commenced, using the low-molecular-weight heparin (LMWH), enoxaparin, subcutaneously twice daily. Postpartum either heparin or warfarin may be used for ongoing anticoagulation, which should continue for 12 weeks.

Clinical comment

Anticoagulants during pregnancy

Warfarin is contraindicated during pregnancy as it is teratogenic and may cause fetal haemorrhage, especially in the third trimester. It may be safely used during breastfeeding, although a small amount is secreted in the milk. Heparin, either unfractionated (UFH) or LMWH, does not cross the placenta so can be safely used in pregnancy. In the non-pregnant state, LMWH is equally effective and safer than UFH in the treatment of VTE. These observations have not yet been fully validated in pregnancy. The major factors in favour of LMWH are:

- significantly decreased incidence of heparin-induced thrombocytopenia
- decreased incidence of osteoporosis
- decreased incidence of bleeding
- significantly higher rate of initial effective anticoagulation
- no requirement for routine monitoring.

'How have I developed DVT?' asks Tegan

You explain to Tegan that the urgency of the caesarean led to the calf compressors not being used, and that this may have contributed to the development of DVT, although you also explain that DVT is a recognised complication of pregnancy and of abdominal surgery. Tegan tells you that she now understands what happened and she is very grateful that Plum is normal and healthy. She also tells you that she and her partner are sure they want no further children and that Peter is arranging to have a vasectomy. You agree that this is a sensible course of action and means that she does not need to be concerned about thromboprophylaxis in future pregnancies or about whether she has contraindications to the COCP.

Clinical pearls

- Whenever an unexpected event or adverse outcome occurs in practice, it is wise to have as full and frank a discussion as possible with all parties concerned soon after the events. This ensures that communication of all important facts is achieved and lessens the chances of subsequent litigation.

References and further reading

Enakpene CA, Omigbodun AO, Arowojolu AO. Perinatal mortality following umbilical cord prolapse. Int J Gynaecol Obstet 2006; 95(1):44–5.

Lagrew DC, Bush MC, McKeown AM, Lagrew NG. Emergent (crash) cesarean delivery: indications and outcomes. Am J Obstet Gynecol 2006; 194(6):1638–43; discussion 1643.

Plumb J, Holwell D. Group B strep: prevention is better than cure. Pract Midwife 2004; 7(3):17–21.

Royal College of Obstetricians and Gynaecologists. Clinical Green-top Guidelines: Thromboprophylaxis During Pregnancy, Labour and after Vaginal Delivery; and Thromboembolic Disease in Pregnancy and the Puerperium; and Group B Streptococcal Disease—Prevention of Early Onset Neonatal. Available online at www.rcog.org.uk..

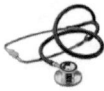

Case 35
Kahlia's baby seems small …

Kahlia is an 18-year-old woman whom you meet for the first time in the antenatal clinic at 33 weeks of pregnancy. She has not booked or had any prior antenatal care apart from an ultrasound at 9 weeks, which was done in a hospital in another town, where she presented with a threatened miscarriage. She had planned to terminate the pregnancy but says she 'did not get around to it and couldn't afford it anyway'. Kahlia comes to the clinic with a supportive female friend with whom she is staying, but says that she no longer has any contact with the baby's father or with her parents, who live in another state. She has just recently moved to your area.

What further history do you take from Kahlia?

Kahlia had regular periods from the age of 13. She became pregnant at the age of 16 and had a termination at 12 weeks. Her periods subsequently became infrequent. Kahlia admits to some heroin use at this time but says she has not used heroin since becoming pregnant; her friend confirms this. She does, however, smoke 20–25 cigarettes a day and uses cannabis on a daily basis. She is on no medications and has no allergies. At the age of 14 she had a ruptured appendix and laparotomy was performed—subsequently she was told she would find it 'very difficult' to become pregnant. For this reason, she says, she has never taken the COCP or used other forms of contraception. She has not had a recent STI check and has never had a Pap smear.

What examination do you make for Kahlia?

Firstly, you perform a general examination. Kahlia is thin, weighing just 45 kg. You observe that she has a number of tattoos and scars on her arms but no recent needle tracks. Her blood pressure is normal and examination of the cardiovascular and respiratory systems shows them to be within normal limits. Examination of the abdomen shows no enlargement of the liver or spleen or other masses apart from the pregnant uterus. The uterine fundal

Recreational drugs and pregnancy

Table 35.1 Effects of recreational drugs in pregnancy

Drugs	Risks in pregnancy	Risks to infant	Management in pregnancy	Remarks
Cannabis	Health risks not clearly established—possible respiratory, mood and psychological problems. Neonate may experience mild withdrawal symptoms in second week of life.	Possible effects on memory and higher cognitive processes in childhood; possible increased hyperactivity and inattention disorders in childhood.	Encourage counselling and psychological treatment for cannabis dependency. Encourage smoking away from infant. No contraindications to breastfeeding.	Cannabis is frequently used in conjunction with tobacco, and cannabis users are often as heavy tobacco users as well. Advice and assistance with quitting tobacco should be offered.
Heroin	Apart from the risks of harm to the mother associated with IV drug use, maternal withdrawal from heroin and other opiates is associated with miscarriage, fetal death in utero, IUGR, preterm labour, and fetal distress in labour.	Withdrawal symptoms in neonates.	Stabilisation on methadone, drug and alcohol counselling, psychosocial support. Women who are stable on methadone should be encouraged to breastfeed.	Infants of heroin-dependent mothers will require close monitoring postnatally, regardless of whether the mother has been stabilised on methadone or not. Close liaison with the social work team is often indicated.
Cocaine	Maternal complications include stroke, seizures, placental abruption, acute myocardial infarction and cardiac arrhythmias. Miscarriage, IUGR, preterm rupture of membranes, preterm labour and stillbirth are increased among cocaine users.	Possible mild withdrawal symptoms in neonates. Necrotising enterocolitis in neonates; possible abnormal behavioural development in infancy.	Pregnant women using cocaine should be advised of the health risks to themselves and their infants. Counselling and psychosocial support should be offered. Early intervention for behavioural and educational problems in cocaine-affected infants have been shown to be beneficial.	Concurrent tobacco use is frequent among cocaine users; it may be difficult to distinguish causation in individual women. Assistance with quitting tobacco should be offered. Women who continue to use cocaine and who wish to breastfeed should be discouraged from breastfeeding for 24 hours following cocaine use.
Amphetamines	Health risks in pregnancy not clearly established. Possible risk of cerebral ischaemia in fetus associated with amphetamine use. Possible IUGR and placental abruption.	Possible mild withdrawal symptoms. Possible agitation and hyperactivity if amphetamines used close to time of birth.	Pregnant women using amphetamines should be advised of health risks to themselves and their infants. Counselling and psychosocial support should be offered.	Women who continue with amphetamine use should be discouraged from breastfeeding for 24 hours following use.

IUGR = intrauterine growth restriction; IV = intravenous.

height is just 29 cm. The baby is lying in the breech position and appears to have little liquor around it. The fetal heart is heard with the hand-held Doppler machine. Kahlia states that she is feeling fetal movements.

Does Kahlia need a vaginal examination?

Kahlia has never had a Pap smear. Although she is well advanced in this pregnancy this may be one of the few opportunities you have to take a Pap smear. You offer to perform it and she consents. You also take endocervical and high and low vaginal swabs for microscopy and culture, as well as a first-catch urine sample for chlamydial and gonococcal PCR.

What investigations do you order for Kahlia, and why?

Kahlia has with her a copy of the ultrasound report from the first hospital so it is clear that her baby is clinically small-for-dates. You order an urgent ultrasound scan for fetal growth, morphology, amniotic fluid index and Doppler measurements of umbilical blood flow. You also order the routine blood and urine tests for antenatal booking visits, which have not yet been performed for Kahlia. While she is still in the clinic you arrange a CTG—the baby's heart rate is within normal limits, reactive, with no decelerations. You arrange to review Kahlia in 2 days' time in the day pregnancy unit. You also arrange for her to talk with the hospital's medical social worker for help with more permanent accommodation and introduction to the local drop-in centre for young single mothers.

> **Intrauterine growth restriction (IUGR) is a major cause of perinatal mortality and morbidity. About 50% of perinatal deaths associated with IUGR are related to underlying chromosomal defects or to intrauterine infections. Other associated factors include low maternal weight (<45 kg pre-pregnancy weight), maternal cigarette smoking or use of other drugs, maternal hypertension, bleeding during pregnancy and a history of previous IUGR.**

How do you manage Kahlia's second consultation?

Kahlia's results are now to hand. There are two features of note. She is positive for hepatitis C virus (HCV). You believe she is unaware of this.

In addition, there is marked slowing of fetal growth with the biparietal diameter and head circumference on the 10th percentile for 32 weeks, abdominal circumference and femur length below this and an EFW of 1400 g. There is a marked drop in liquor volume, with an AFI of 5.1 and Doppler scans show absent end-diastolic flow. However, detailed scanning shows no anatomical abnormality. Kahlia also tells you that the baby is moving much less than previously.

What is the immediate management for Kahlia?

A CTG is performed and this shows a non-reassuring trace. Your consultant decides that immediate delivery is indicated and arrangements are made for caesarean section. A baby girl weighing 1380 g is delivered in fair condition, with Apgar scores of 3 at 1 minute and 7 at 5 minutes. The infant is transferred to the care of the paediatricians.

What are your ongoing concerns for Kahlia?

Kahlia needs a detailed consultation to explain the significance and long-term implications of the finding of HCV antibodies on routine screening. This will include the information that HCV transmission has not been shown to be reduced by delivery by means of caesarean section. Kahlia's daughter should be tested for HCV at 18 months of age, when transplacental antibodies will have disappeared from the infant's blood. Mother-to-child transmission is uncommon during delivery and breastfeeding is not contraindicated. Kahlia requires referral to the sexual health clinic for ongoing management and follow-up of her own HCV status and you arrange this while she is in the postnatal ward. She is also given a referral to the social worker attached to your maternity unit for assistance with housing, financial entitlements and other support. In addition, before discharge you discuss contraception and the need for safe sexual practices in depth with her.

Clinical pearls

- Hepatitis C infection is increasing in incidence among Australian women. Antenatal screening should routinely include screening for HCV infection—there are implications not only for the woman but also for her child.

References and further reading

Centers for Disease Control and Prevention; Workowski KA, Berman SM. Sexually transmitted diseases treatment guidelines, 2006. MMWR Recomm Rep 2006; 55(RR-11):1–94.

Clarke A, Kulasegaram R. Hepatitis C transmission—where are we now? Int J STD AIDS 2006; 17(2):74–80; quiz 80.

Giles ML, Garland SM, Grover SR, Lewin SM, Hellard ME. Impact of an education campaign on management in pregnancy of women infected with a blood-borne virus. Med J Aust 2006; 184(8):389–92.

Society of Obstetricians and Gynaecologists of Canada. Clinical Practice Guidelines:The Reproductive Care of Women Living with Hepatitis C Infection. Available online at www.socg.org.

Zuccotti GV, Salvini F, Farina F, Agostoni C, Riva E, Giovannini M. Longitudinal long-term follow-up study of children with vertically acquired hepatitis C virus infection. J Int Med Res 2006; 34(2):215–22.

Part 4
Clinical Cases in Gynaecology

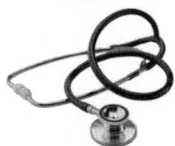

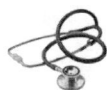

Case 36
Rebecca presents with acute abdominal pain ...

You are working in the emergency department of a country hospital when you are called early one Sunday morning to see Rebecca, a 20-year-old woman who has presented complaining of severe lower abdominal pain. When you arrive you find Rebecca lying on her left side on a bed in a cubicle, her legs drawn up and very distressed by the pain. Vital signs have already been recorded by the nursing staff—blood pressure 100/80 mmHg, pulse 100 bpm, temperature 39.5°C.

What is your immediate management of Rebecca?

You explain to Rebecca that she will be given pain relief very shortly but that you must first get some idea of the cause of her problem. You take a short but relevant history: the pain has been present for 24 hours but has increased greatly since midnight. It has always been in the lower abdomen but is much worse on the right side. She has never had a similar pain. She has not had her appendix removed or any other abdominal surgery. Her periods have been a bit irregular lately, the last one being about 5 weeks ago.

'How long have they been irregular?', you ask. Rebecca then tells you that she had a termination of pregnancy 4 months ago and was also treated for chlamydia—cycles have since been irregular and short with episodes of spotting in between. The clinic where she had the termination has given her a prescription for the oral contraceptive pill but because of the irregular bleeding she has not yet commenced this. She is still with the same partner and they use condoms 'most of the time'. She agrees that she could possibly be pregnant again. There have been no urinary or bowel symptoms.

What examination do you now make?

A quick general physical examination reveals nothing remarkable although Rebecca is clearly very distressed by the pain. On palpating her abdomen you find marked tenderness in the right lower quadrant with rebound and guarding—Rebecca pushes your hand away. In the left lower quadrant there is also tenderness on palpation but no guarding or rebound tenderness. You ask Rebecca if she could produce a urine specimen—she provides a sample for pregnancy testing and a midstream urine (MSU) sample for microscopy and culture. A rapidly performed commercial kit pregnancy test is negative.

> Commercial pregnancy tests are quantitative, with a sensitivity equivalent to a blood concentration of beta-human chorionic gonadotrophin (β-HCG) of 50 IU/L. Tests will become positive about the time of the first missed period, usually 14 days postconception.

Should you perform a vaginal examination for Rebecca?

Yes. This is essential in making a diagnosis with this presentation. Gently passing a speculum, you examine the cervix, which is inflamed with a yellowish discharge coming from the os. You take swabs from the endocervix for general microscopy and culture, and chlamydial and gonococcal screening. Rebecca reports having had a normal Pap smear result 6 months previously.

Bimanual vaginal examination elicits excruciating tenderness in the right fornix with an impression of fullness in the adnexae, although you do not persist with the examination because of the pain it is clearly causing. There

Clinical picture of acute pelvic infection

- Most common presentation is in a young, sexually active woman
- Most common initiating cause is a sexually transmitted infection (STI) (in Australia, chlamydial infection is the most common followed by gonorrhoea)
- May follow vaginal delivery or a gynaecological operation (e.g. termination of pregnancy, endometrial sampling, intrauterine contraceptive device insertion)
- Associated with severe lower abdominal pain and peritonism, usually bilateral but may be more marked on one side
- Pyrexia—usually the temperature is significantly raised
- Vaginal examination reveals severe tenderness in one or both lateral fornices and cervical excitation

is also tenderness in the left fornix and over the body of the uterus itself, which does not feel enlarged, and severe tenderness on gently moving the cervix. You make a clinical diagnosis of acute pelvic infection.

What is your ongoing management in this case?

Rebecca is given IM pethidine for pain, an intravenous line is established, blood is taken for a full blood count (FBC) and rapid plasma reagin (RPR; syphilis screening), and she is commenced on cefoxitin IV 6-hourly and doxycycline 100 mg orally 12-hourly. Arrangements are made to admit her to the ward.

Treatment regimens for acute pelvic infection

- Cefoxitin or cefotetan IV plus doxycycline orally *or*
- Ceftriaxone or cefotaxime IV plus metronidazole plus doxycycline *or*
- Amoxycillin/potassium clavulanate IV plus metronidazole plus doxycycline *or*
- Clindamycin plus gentamicin
- If no response in 24–36 hours, reconsider diagnosis or complication of pelvic inflammatory disease (PID) (e.g. pelvic abscess)
- Full STI screen should be performed on all women presenting with PID

The following day you see Rebecca on your ward round. She is now sitting up in bed, feeling much better, although she still has some abdominal pain. She no longer requires narcotic analgesia. Her temperature has settled to 37.6°C and her pulse rate to 80 bpm. Palpation of her abdomen produces some tenderness but no rebound or guarding. Rebecca is able to tolerate a normal diet.

What further care does Rebecca need?

You check the results of the tests you ordered the previous day and find that Rebecca's FBC showed a marked leucocytosis with a white cell count of 17×10^9/L with a neutrophilia, raised erythrocyte sedimentation rate (ESR) and C-reactive protein, but that her haemoglobin and red blood cell measurements are within normal limits. The urinary chlamydia PCR test is positive, and urine microscopy shows small numbers of leucocytes and epithelial cells only. Swabs show a growth of *Streptococcus faecalis*.

These results are consistent with your diagnosis of acute pelvic infection, probably initiated by a new chlamydial infection on a background of mild endometritis following termination of pregnancy. You explain the diagnosis to Rebecca, emphasising the need for adequate antibiotic treatment, rest and abstinence from sexual activity until she is better, if possible the tracing and treatment of sexual contacts, and the importance of safe sex in the future. You explain that acute infection in the fallopian tubes can lead to infertility or ectopic pregnancy at a later date when she does actually want to become pregnant. Rebecca should commence her oral contraceptive pill at the time of her next period but should also use condoms unless or until she is certain that she and her partner are in a monogamous relationship.

Clinical pearls

Distinguishing acute PID from appendicitis

- In PID, pain always starts in the lower abdomen and is generally bilateral; in appendicitis, pain starts around the umbilicus or in the upper abdomen, later becoming unilateral.
- Women have a higher temperature in PID.
- Cervical excitation and tenderness in both fornices is characteristic of PID, although pain may predominate on one side.
- Nausea and anorexia is characteristic of appendicitis.
- Remember pregnancy can coexist with PID or appendicitis!
- Do not let a woman of reproductive age languish without a diagnosis—laparoscopy must be performed early if empirical therapy is not successful.

References and further reading

Chen MY, Pan Y, Britt H et al. Trends in clinical encounters for pelvic inflammatory disease and epididymitis in a national sample of Australian general practices. Int J STD AIDS 2006; 17(6):384–6.

Cole E, Lynch A, Cugnoni H. Assessment of the patient with acute abdominal pain. Nurs Stand 2006; 20(38):56–61.

Manavi K. A review of infection with Chlamydia trachomatis. Best Pract Res Clin Obstet Gynaecol 2006; August 22. (E-publication ahead of printing.)

Royal College of Obstetricians and Gynaecologists, Clinical Green-top Guidelines: Management of Acute Pelvic Inflammatory Disease. Available online at www.rcog.org.uk.

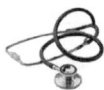

Case 37
Vicky has postmenopausal bleeding …

In the gynaecology outpatients' department you see for the first time a 57-year-old woman, Vicky. Vicky has been referred urgently by her general practitioner, Dr Case, because she presented to her with an episode of vaginal bleeding approximately 18 months after her last apparent menstrual period. Dr Case has performed a Pap smear and organised a transvaginal pelvic ultrasound—the results of these investigations are not to hand at the time when you first see Vicky.

You take a detailed gynaecological and full medical history from Vicky. She tells you that there has been only one episode of bleeding, which occurred after she had been helping her daughter move a wardrobe in her new house, in preparation for the arrival of Vicky's first grandchild. Vicky says she only went to see Dr Case because the bleeding made her realise that she had not had a Pap smear for some time—'some time' turned out to be 5 years. Vicky is sure it was just the heavy lifting that caused the bleeding. She is also sure the referral to hospital is unnecessary and she hopes there won't be any need for any further investigations because her daughter's baby is due any day now.

Vicky began her periods at age 14; they were always heavy and often irregular, especially in the years before her menopause. She had a dilatation and curettage performed in her late 40s, but this showed nothing abnormal. She has had only one pregnancy, her daughter, conceived after 5 years of marriage; she would have liked more children, but 'it just didn't happen'.

Vicky is a type 2 diabetic, diagnosed 5 years ago. She tries to stick to a good diet but admits she finds it difficult and freely agrees she is overweight at 102 kg. She takes metformin for diabetic control and also states that she has high blood pressure. Dr Case has listed amlodipine among her medications. Vicky has a family history of heart disease and diabetes on both sides. Her mother died from breast cancer in her 60s and Vicky says she herself is careful to have regular mammograms—more careful than she is about her Pap smears. Vicky has had a cholecystectomy and appendicectomy in the past and her one child was born by caesarean section and weighed 4530 g.

General physical examination shows a woman of late middle age who is definitely obese. Her blood pressure is 130/90 mmHg. Examination of the cardiovascular system and abdomen is unremarkable, although obesity limits the value of abdominal palpation.

At this point the results of Vicky's Pap smear and pelvic ultrasound reach you by fax. The Pap smear is reported as showing normal squamous cells but there are 'endometrial cells present suggestive of endometrial adenocarcinoma'. The ultrasound scan shows a uterus of normal size (8 cm in length) with a thickened endometrium—the endometrial stripe measures 13 mm. The ovaries are small and no cysts or other abnormalities are visualised.

Does Vicky need a further vaginal examination?

There is no need to perform another vaginal examination for Vicky at this point. You have all the information you need from the general practitioner's letter and the ultrasound scan report. You note from Dr Case's letter that she observed a degree of atrophic vaginitis at the time of performing the Pap smear. Possibly this was, in fact, the source of the vaginal bleeding. However, you must explain the implications of the findings to Vicky, the very probable diagnosis of endometrial cancer and what this will entail.

Atrophic vaginitis is the most common cause of postmenopausal bleeding. However, all women presenting with postmenopausal bleeding, even when atrophic vaginitis is present, must be investigated fully to exclude endometrial cancer.

What information do you now give Vicky?

The Pap smear, you tell her, when she is again dressed and sitting in the consulting room, shows some abnormal cells that have come from the lining of the womb. The ultrasound also shows some thickening of that lining. The good news is that she has come along early. If cancer is confirmed, this is a type of cancer with a very good outlook, especially when found early. It is more common in women who have no or few children and women who are diabetic, so Vicky fits the bill on all counts.

Vicky is more philosophical about this than you had expected. 'Of course', she says, 'I will come for whatever treatment I need. What happens next?', she wants to know.

What further investigations and treatment are likely to be offered to Vicky?

She will need a hysteroscopy, you explain, to completely visualise the inside of the uterus, and an examination under anaesthesia, as well as curettage of the endometrium and pathological examination to make an accurate diagnosis. This will be done in conjunction with one of the gynaecological oncologists who attends the hospital.

Predisposing factors to endometrial cancer

- Age—more common in older women who are either peri- or postmenopausal
- History of early onset of menarche, late menopause
- Obesity
- Type 2 diabetes mellitus
- Endometrial hyperplasia with atypia
- Unopposed exogenous oestrogen therapy
- Polycystic ovarian syndrome
- Tamoxifen therapy
- Western lifestyle possibly contributes

Note: Women who have used the combined oral contraceptive pill (COCP) for at least 2 years have a 40% reduction in the incidence of endometrial cancer.

Clinical comment

Stages of endometrial cancer

Staging is surgical, with total abdominal hysterectomy and bilateral salpingo-oophorectomy (TAH/BSO) performed through a midline incision, peritoneal washings for cytology and selective pelvic lymph node sampling.

Stage	Description
I	Cancer remains in the body of the uterus
IA	Cancer is in the endometrium only
IB	Cancer has invaded less than half of the thickness of the myometrium
IC	Cancer has extended to more than half of the thickness of the myometrium
II	The tumour has extended to the cervix
III	The tumour has spread beyond the uterus but is still in the pelvic area
IV	There is more distant spread of the cancer

Current treatment of endometrial cancer is usually by a combination of surgery and radiotherapy. If the lesion is confined to the inner half of the uterus and is histologically well differentiated, TAH/BSO is sufficient treatment. Higher stages and grades will need pelvic radiotherapy after surgery. Some histological types, including small cell and clear cell adenocarcinoma, are high risk. These cases usually require chemotherapy.

Table 37.1 Five-year survival rates for endometrial cancer

Stage	5-year survival rate
I	90%
II	70–85%
III	50%
IV	10–30%

Clinical pearls

- All women presenting with a history of postmenopausal bleeding, however slight, should have endometrial cancer excluded.
- A physical examination, Pap smear and ultrasound scan measuring the endometrial thickness should always be performed—if the endometrium is clearly visualised and measures less than 5 mm in thickness, further investigation may not be needed; however, in many cases hysteroscopy and curettage will be appropriate.

References and further reading

Kitchener H. Management of endometrial cancer. Eur J Surg Oncol 2006; 32(8):838–43.

O'Connor V, Kovacs G, eds. Obstetrics, Gynaecology and Women's Health. Melbourne: Cambridge University Press, 2003:568–70.

Romer T. Hormone replacement therapy and bleeding disorders. Gynecol Endocrinol 2006; 22(3):140–4.

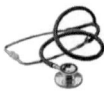

Case 38
Rani has an ovarian cyst …

Rani is a 17-year-old teenager whom you are asked to see urgently at the emergency department where she has presented with acute abdominal pain, having been sent into hospital by her general practitioner.

When you arrive in the cubicle Rani lies curled on her side and is clearly distressed. Her vital signs have already been taken: blood pressure 110/70 mmHg, pulse rate 100 bpm, temperature 37.0°C.

What are your first steps?

You take a short history from Rani. Her mother, who is present and anxious, does not speak much English but attempts to answer all your questions instead of her daughter.

> It is important to take the history from the patient herself. She is legally able to give consent for herself and in this case can speak English perfectly.

How do you handle this situation?

You politely but firmly ask the mother to sit next to her daughter and tell her you will ask questions of Rani alone.

Rani tells you she has had some vague lower abdominal pain for a few months. She has seen her general practitioner, who did not find anything wrong on abdominal examination. An abdominal ultrasound has been ordered but has not yet been performed. Today she experienced the sudden severe onset of right iliac fossa pain, somewhat like the vague pains she has been having but much worse. She vomited once and now feels a bit nauseous and not hungry. Her menstrual cycle is regular, last menstrual period (LMP)

2 weeks previously, she has never been on the COCP, takes no medications and has no allergies. She has no serious medical problems and has never had any surgery. There are no urinary or bowel symptoms.

Do you examine Rani in her mother's presence?

It is advisable to take a sexual history from Rani without her mother present in view of her age. It would be appropriate to ask her mother to sit outside while you examine Rani.

With her mother out of earshot you gently inquire whether Rani is sexually active. She denies this, is quite sure of the date of her LMP and has no other health problems of note.

A short general examination shows no signs of anaemia and confirms Rani's tachycardia. You ask Rani to lie on her back and extend her legs—she has difficulty doing this and finds the pain is less with her legs flexed. Inspection of the abdomen reveals no obvious distension or masses. Palpation reveals acute tenderness in the right lower quadrant with guarding and rebound tenderness. There is minimal tenderness in the left lower quadrant and none in the upper abdomen; the liver and spleen are not palpable and there is no tenderness over the renal angles.

Do you perform a vaginal examination for Rani?

No. Rani has never been sexually active nor used tampons. As well, vaginal examination may be culturally inappropriate. As already noted, vaginal examination should not be performed in a virgin. However, it is clear that Rani has an acute problem in the right side of her pelvis. In a young woman with similar symptoms, who has become sexually active, vaginal examination will be helpful in establishing a diagnosis and should be performed.

What investigations should be performed?

FBC, MSU, urea and electrolytes, and a transabdominal ultrasound scan should be performed. You order intravenous fluids to help fill the bladder prior to the ultrasound scan. You also perform a urine β-HCG test, which is negative.

You prescribe pethidine and metoclopramide for Rani and keep her fasting.

Differential diagnosis of acute right-sided lower abdominal pain in a young woman

- Appendicitis
- PID
- Ectopic pregnancy
- Complications of ovarian tumours (usually cysts)

The FBC shows normal haemoglobin and platelet levels, with a slightly raised white cell count (9×10^9/L) and ESR. Serum electrolytes are in the normal range.

The ultrasound scan shows a normal-sized uterus deviated to the left by the presence of a 6 cm diameter cyst in the right adnexae. There is a considerable amount of fluid in the pouch of Douglas. The cyst contains solid material and has the appearance of a dermoid cyst. The left ovary appears normal. You make a provisional diagnosis of a leaking right ovarian cyst and prepare Rani for surgery.

You assist your consultant with laparoscopy, at which your diagnosis is confirmed. There is a quantity of sebaceous material in the pouch of Douglas, and the cyst has undergone torsion. There are a number of fibrinous adhesions around the right tube and ovary. It is decided to proceed to a laparotomy, at which the cyst is untwisted, and ovarian cystectomy, conserving a portion of viable normal ovary, is performed. The cyst is noted to contain hair as well as more sebaceous material. The left ovary is inspected and appears entirely normal.

> Simple cysts in young women can usually be treated laparoscopically but when complications have occurred or there is any possibility of malignancy, laparotomy may be the safer option.

Subsequent histology confirms a benign dermoid cyst. You reassure Rani and her parents that the remaining ovarian tissue is normal and that Rani's ultimate reproductive functioning will not be compromised.

Clinical comment

Complications of ovarian cysts include torsion, haemorrhage into cyst, leaking of cyst contents, infection and adhesions to adjacent organs.

Classification of ovarian cysts

- Physiological—follicular or luteal—normally not larger than 6 cm diameter, can be watched on ultrasound, if causing symptoms ovarian function can be suppressed with COCP
- Benign epithelial tumours—serous cystadenoma, mucinous (pseudomucinous) cystadenoma, endometrioid cystadenoma, Brenner tumour
- Benign germ cell tumours—dermoid cyst, mature teratoma
- Benign sex cord stromal tumours
- Theca cell tumours—fibroma, Sertoli-Leydig cell tumour
- Borderline
- Malignant

Clinical pearls

- Analgesia should not be administered to patients with unexplained abdominal pain until a working diagnosis has been reached and appropriate investigations instigated.
- It is prudent to consider the possibility of pregnancy in every young woman presenting with abdominal symptoms; pregnancy is easily and accurately excluded as a cause of the presentation with urine β-HCG testing. This is true even when pregnancy seems unlikely from the history and social circumstances of the woman. It is essential that pregnancy not be missed in any significant presentation involving the abdomen.

References and further reading

Carter J, Pather S, Abdel-Hadi M et al. Not all ovarian cysts in young women are benign: a case series and review of the management of complex adnexal masses in young women. Aust N Z J Obstet Gynaecol 2006; 46(4):350–5.

O'Connor V, Kovacs G, eds. Obstetrics, Gynaecology and Women's Health. Melbourne: Cambridge University Press, 2003:570–4.

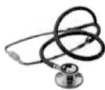

Case 39
Sharon is bleeding in early pregnancy …

Late one Saturday evening you are called to the emergency department to see Sharon, who is a 29-year-old primigravida. Sharon has been trying to conceive for about 6 months. A week ago she performed a home pregnancy test, which was positive. She and her partner Gary have been very excited about this. However, this evening she has experienced some crampy lower abdominal pain and spotting and is now very concerned and frightened.

What history do you need to take from Sharon?

You take a short history from Sharon. Her LMP was 7 weeks ago, but her cycles are irregular, anything from 4 to 6 weeks in length. She has seen her general practitioner, who also confirmed the pregnancy by urinary β-HCG testing and has ordered a pelvic ultrasound for help with dating, but Sharon has not yet had this scan.

Sharon is otherwise in good health with no relevant medical or surgical history, in particular no history of STIs. She has never been on the oral contraceptive pill and she stopped smoking completely 9 months ago. She takes no medications apart from folic acid and has no allergies. Her last Pap smear was a year ago and the report was normal.

What physical examination is necessary in Sharon's case?

Apart from a brief general examination and measurement of blood pressure, pulse and temperature, Sharon should have both abdominal and vaginal examinations performed.

Sharon's vital signs are all within normal limits. Abdominal inspection is unremarkable and palpation simply shows some mild central lower abdominal tenderness. There is no guarding or rebound tenderness, no tenderness elsewhere in the abdomen and no uterine enlargement or other masses.

Vaginal examination reveals a cervix that is closed on inspection through a speculum, with some dark blood visible at the os. Bimanual palpation shows a bulky, soft, slightly tender uterus.

What is your clinical diagnosis and what investigations are indicated at this point?

Clinically Sharon has a threatened miscarriage—she is known to be pregnant with some bleeding and the cervix is closed. However, there has not been any confirmation so far that her pregnancy is in the uterus and the possibility of an ectopic pregnancy should not be overlooked. An ultrasound scan may be helpful in making a definite diagnosis.

You are able to perform a transvaginal ultrasound scan using the portable machine in the emergency department. This shows a gestational sac within the uterus and a fetal pole of 5 mm crown–rump length, indicating a gestational age of just 6 weeks, however, you are unable to demonstrate a beating fetal heart. You explain to Sharon and Gary that the pregnancy is in the right site, you show them the fetus explaining how small it is and that it is often not possible to detect a fetal heart until the pregnancy is several more days advanced. Since Sharon's cycles are irregular it is possible that she has a continuing pregnancy and that the fetal heart will become detectable on ultrasound within days. You explain to the couple that unexplained slight bleeding in early pregnancy is not uncommon and may settle spontaneously, the pregnancy continuing normally thereafter. However, there is also the possibility, since there is bleeding from within the uterus, that she may miscarry.

Since Sharon's general physical state is satisfactory you advise her to go home and tell her that while rest has not been shown to have a preventive effect from the point of view of the pregnancy, she may feel better in herself by taking some time off work and resting over a few days until all bleeding ceases. You also advise her to avoid sexual intercourse until bleeding settles. After taking blood for an FBC, quantitative β-HCG levels and blood group and Rhesus status, you arrange for her to be seen in the early pregnancy clinic the following Monday for ongoing assessment of her pregnancy and advise her to continue taking folic acid. She appears reassured by your advice.

However, early on Sunday morning you are called back to the emergency department to see Sharon again. For the past hour she has been bleeding more heavily, she now has severe lower abdominal pain and feels 'weak and sweaty'.

On examination Sharon looks pale and is shivering. Her pulse is 100 bpm, blood pressure 90/50 mmHg and temperature 36.8°C. Abdominal examination now shows increased central tenderness above the pubic symphysis. Speculum examination shows an open cervix with placental tissue in the os accompanied by brisk bright red bleeding.

What is your management?

Products of conception in the cervical canal holding the cervix open can cause a degree of shock disproportionate to the amount of blood lost. Products of conception should be removed with sponge forceps or digitally using sterile gloves. Removal of all visible products of conception can greatly improve the clinical situation.

With sponge forceps you grasp the placental tissue and remove it. Bleeding, however, continues so you administer ergometrine 0.5 mg IM. You also commence Sharon on intravenous fluids.

You explain to Sharon that she has, in fact, miscarried and passed at least part of the pregnancy. You add that this is disappointing but unfortunately miscarriage is quite common, occurring in about 15% of pregnancies. However, most women experiencing miscarriage in a first pregnancy, you tell her, go on to have a normal pregnancy on the second occasion.

'What causes the miscarriage?' Gary asks

In most miscarriages the reason is unknown, although it is known that a high proportion of spontaneously aborted embryos have chromosomal abnormalities. Examination of the products of conception does not usually help in determining the cause of the miscarriage in the individual case.

Sharon is still bleeding moderately despite the administration of ergometrine. What is your further management?

You recommend to Sharon that she undergo removal of any remaining tissue from within the uterus under a general anaesthetic. This will stop bleeding and reassure her that the miscarriage is complete. She agrees to this and later that morning has suction curettage performed. The results of her blood tests from the previous evening are available—Sharon's haemoglobin level at that time was 131 g/L, and her blood group is A Rhesus positive. Sharon does not require anti-D prophylaxis.

Before discharge home later that day you arrange for Sharon to see her own general practitioner during the week. You tell her that her next period should start within 4–6 weeks following the miscarriage. She asks whether she can then try again to become pregnant and you reassure her about this, advising her that there is no increased risk of miscarriage in her next pregnancy. You advise her to continue with folate supplements as she has been doing.

Table 39.1 Types of miscarriage and their characteristics

Type of miscarriage	Bleeding	Pain	Clinical findings
Threatened	Slight	None	Cervix closed, uterus size = dates
Inevitable	Moderate to heavy	Moderate to severe	Cervix open, no tissue seen
Incomplete	Moderate to heavy	Moderate to severe	Cervix open, tissue seen
Complete	Slight or none	Settling or none	Cervix open or closed, tissue passed
Missed	Slight or none	None	Cervix closed, uterus small for dates

Note: All types of miscarriage may be complicated by infection.

Clinical pearls

- Expectant management is safe for women experiencing miscarriage if bleeding is slight to moderate and pain is tolerable—this will be most women presenting. Surgical evacuation of the uterus is indicated for heavy bleeding, although on occasion it may also be requested by women.

References and further reading

Chamberlain G, Steer P, eds. Turnbull's Obstetrics. 3rd edn. London: Churchill Livingstone, 2001:117–29.

Christiansen OB. Evidence-based investigations and treatments of recurrent pregnancy loss. Curr Opin Obstet Gynecol 2006; 18(3):304–12.

Rai R, Regan L. Recurrent miscarriage. Lancet 2006; 368(9535):601–11.

Royal College of Obstetricians and Gynaecologists. Clinical Green-top Guidelines: The Investigation and Treatment of Recurrent Pregnancy Loss. Available online at www.rcog.org.uk.

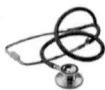

Case 40
Angie presents with an ectopic pregnancy …

You are called urgently to the emergency department to see Angie, a 25-year-old woman who has presented with severe left-sided lower abdominal pain. On arrival you find that Angie's observations have already been taken by nursing staff—pulse 100 bpm, blood pressure 90/60 mmHg, temperature 36.8°C. Angie is lying with her legs drawn up looking pale and distressed. She is able to tell you that the pain began during sexual intercourse about 1 hour previously. She does remember experiencing some similar but very mild pain the previous day.

What is your overriding concern in your assessment of Angie?

She may have an ectopic pregnancy that has ruptured or is about to rupture with the risk of life-threatening intra-abdominal haemorrhage.

Quickly you take a short relevant history from Angie. Her LMP was 6 weeks previously. Her cycles are irregular and 6 weeks is not unusual for her. She had some spotting the previous day, which she thought was the start of a period but no more has followed. Although not wishing to be pregnant she has had unprotected sex with two partners during the past month. She has a 6-year-old son born by caesarean section.

What is your next step?

Angie is able to produce a urine specimen with the help of nursing staff and while this is being tested you examine her. She is pale and sweating. Inspection shows some lower abdominal distension. On palpation the abdomen is rigid in the left lower quadrant, very tender with rebound tenderness when you remove your hand. The nursing staff now report that Angie's urine pregnancy test is positive.

On the basis of this information you make a tentative diagnosis of ruptured ectopic pregnancy. Angie's clinical condition is such that urgent surgical intervention is needed. You explain to Angie that you believe she has an ectopic pregnancy, probably in her left tube, which has ruptured. You will be calling in urgently a senior colleague to operate as well as anaesthetic and nursing staff. You proceed at once to insert a wide-bore intravenous cannula for Angie and take blood for an FBC, group and cross-match of two units of whole blood. You commence Angie on a litre of Hartmann's solution to run in rapidly. You gain consent from Angie for a laparoscopy and/or laparotomy, explaining that if possible the procedure will be done by laparoscopy but that her condition may make it necessary to proceed to laparotomy. You explain that if a tubal pregnancy is present and bleeding, then part or all of the tube may need to be removed. Your consultant will also inspect the other tube and discuss the findings with Angie postoperatively.

Upon arrival in the operating theatre Angie's blood pressure has dropped to 80/50 mmHg and her lower abdomen is more distended. The surgeon makes the decision to proceed at once to laparotomy, at which you assist. He finds more than 1 L of fresh blood and clots in the pelvis. There is free bleeding from a distended and ruptured portion of the left fallopian tube and a small amount of placental tissue protruding from the tube. The distal end of the tube is stuck to the ovary and the right tube also shows signs of chronic infection. A partial salpingectomy is performed, excising the portion of tube containing the ectopic pregnancy, and haemostasis is achieved satisfactorily. Angie's condition improves and stabilises with intravenous fluids, and although blood is available it is not used.

The following day you see Angie on your ward round. *'What are my chances of future pregnancy?'* she asks

Angie had definite evidence at laparotomy of chronic pelvic infection. She has had swabs taken from both tubes at the time of surgery and you have prescribed antibiotics (tinidazole and doxycycline) to cover the postoperative period pending microbiological reports. Angie then admits to having been treated twice in the past 2 years for chlamydial infections. You explain that the condition of her tubes plus the removal of part of the left one does mean that she may have difficulty conceiving again and that there is an increased risk of any pregnancy that does occur being an ectopic again. If she does experience difficulty conceiving and wishes to proceed with treatment, then in-vitro fertilisation is the procedure most likely to be successful.

She then says that she has a friend who had an ectopic pregnancy who was treated laparoscopically. 'Why couldn't I have been done the same way and so ended up with a smaller, less painful scar?'

What is your response to this question?

Angie's condition had become life-threatening because the ectopic pregnancy had ruptured the fallopian tube, causing severe intraperitoneal haemorrhage. Often ectopic pregnancy is diagnosed when a woman known to be pregnant presents with an ultrasound report showing an empty uterus—there may or may not be ultrasound evidence of the pregnancy developing in one or other tube. Ectopic pregnancy may also present with mild lower abdominal pain in a woman known to be in early pregnancy—the pain is due to slight bleeding irritating the peritoneal surface. There may also be slight vaginal bleeding, as in Angie's case, as fluctuating progesterone levels from developing placental tissue act upon the decidualised endometrium. Where the woman's condition is stable, laparoscopy to confirm the diagnosis and provide treatment is the preferred option.

Clinical comment

Bleeding in early pregnancy—distinguishing ectopic pregnancy from miscarriage

Vaginal bleeding associated with ectopic pregnancy tends to be slight and intermittent, and pain is constant and most severe on the side on which the ectopic pregnancy is located. Bleeding associated with miscarriage is frequently moderate in amount but may be severe, especially with inevitable or incomplete miscarriage; pain is central and colicky. Quantitative β-HCG levels may be measured in cases where the woman is stable, and when a level of >1000 U is reached; a fetal pole should be visible on transvaginal ultrasound. In a continuing intrauterine pregnancy, β-HCG levels should double every 48 hours.

When the diagnosis of ectopic pregnancy is made early in pregnancy and the fallopian tube has not ruptured, medical treatment with methotrexate may bring about absorption and resolution of the pregnancy without the need for surgical intervention. However, the methotrexate must be given under close medical supervision and surgery proceeded to if pain supervenes or serum β-HCG levels do not fall by at least 15% within 4 days. Levels should be followed until they become negative.

Clinical pearls

- Ectopic pregnancy should be considered as a possible diagnosis in every woman presenting with abdominal pain.
- Only early ectopic pregnancy with minimal signs and symptoms is suitable for management with methotrexate; patients with features of peritonism or an unstable cardiovascular status require surgical treatment.

References and further reading

Crossman SH. The challenge of pelvic inflammatory disease. Am Fam Physician 2006; 73(5):859–64.

Gray-Swain MR, Peipert JF. Pelvic inflammatory disease in adolescents. Curr Opin Obstet Gynecol 2006; 18(5):503–10.

Ramakrishnan K, Scheid DC. Ectopic pregnancy: expectant management of immediate surgery? J Fam Pract 2006; 55(6):517–22.

Ramakrishnan K, Scheid DC. Ectopic pregnancy: forget the 'classic presentation' if you want to catch it sooner. J Fam Pract 2006; 55(5):388–95.

Royal College of Obstetricians and Gynaecologists. Clinical Green-top Guidelines: Management of Tubal Pregnancy. Available online at www.rcog.org.uk.

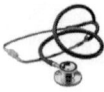

Case 41
Sandra is bothered by 'leaking' …

Sandra is a 54-year-old woman who has noticed worsening urinary incontinence for the last 3 years. She has also noticed a 'lump' protruding through her vagina, which is beginning to bother her. Initially she noticed the lump while taking a shower, and was frightened she may have found a cancer. Then she remembered that her mother had had a prolapse and realised that this was probably what was happening to her. At first it didn't bother her too much, but it is now present on most days and although not painful, is certainly uncomfortable. Sandra is fond of gardening and the lump is particularly bad after spending a day lifting, carrying and digging in the garden. She has been putting up with both the incontinence and the prolapse, but has now decided enough is enough and has come to the gynaecology outpatients department with a referral from her general practitioner to 'have it all fixed'.

Sandra says that a friend of hers has had a new tape operation and it cured her incontinence.

> *'I just want that tape operation, doctor, to fix everything up. My friend went into hospital for one day and she said it was marvellous'*, Sandra says

You agree with Sandra that some of the new operations for particular forms of incontinence are indeed marvellous, but that perhaps it would be better to spend a bit of time discussing her problems first. You explain that as she seems to have both urinary incontinence and a prolapse, the situation may be a little more complicated than it was for her friend. You begin by asking her a few questions about her incontinence.

Firstly, when does she lose urine?

'When I cough and sneeze mainly, and sometimes if I run quickly or run up the steps at home.'

How long has this been happening?

'About 3 or 4 years—it seems to have worsened since I went through the menopause when I was 49.'

What further questions should be asked?

Sandra should be asked several direct questions:

- 'Do you ever need to pass urine in a hurry, or sometimes not make it to the toilet and have an accident?'—'Yes, this does happen sometimes but not often.'
- 'Do you need to get up at night to go to the toilet?'—'Once or twice a night.'
- 'Do you need to wear any continence protection pads?'—'Yes, I buy them from the supermarket and I need to use them every day.'
- 'Do you have urinary frequency, burning or stinging when you pass urine, blood in the urine, or bowel problems?'—Sandra answers no to all these.

Clinical comment

- There are four types of incontinence in women—true incontinence (usually due to a urinary fistula—rare), overflow incontinence (less common than in men as it occurs with urinary obstruction), urinary stress incontinence and urinary urge incontinence.
- The latter two are the most important and are common. Stress incontinence is more common than urge incontinence, but most women presenting have features of both—mixed incontinence.
- Stress incontinence is a symptom. It may be due to a hypermobile urethra, which occurs as a result of childbirth and ageing, or more rarely a urinary sphincter mechanism deficiency. If this is confirmed on urodynamic studies, the diagnosis is called 'urodynamic stress incontinence' (previously known as 'genuine stress incontinence').
- Urge incontinence may be secondary to poor bladder habits, but can also be due to 'detrusor overactivity' (previously known as 'detrusor instability'), where the bladder contracts and empties at abnormally low volumes of urine and cannot be controlled by conscious effort.

What history do you take from Sandra relevant to her complaints of prolapse?

Sandra tells you that she has noticed this for the past 3 or 4 years and it is quite uncomfortable. There is no history of postmenopausal bleeding or discharge, although the lump does rub on her underwear, causing local irritation. She has four children, all born vaginally; the first baby being a forceps delivery. She is sexually active but the prolapse does make intercourse slightly uncomfortable, and her vagina feels dry unless she uses lubrication. She is otherwise healthy and well; in particular, she is not obese, does not have any chronic lung conditions, and is on no medication. Her last Pap smear was about 3 years ago and her last mammogram 1 year ago.

What examination do you make for Sandra?

You perform a general examination and then an abdominal examination: these are unremarkable. You then carry out a vaginal examination. Her external genitalia appear normal. You perform a Sims' speculum examination in the left lateral position. You can demonstrate a moderate cystocele when you ask her to 'bear down'. Elevating the cystocele with a pair of sponge-holding forceps, you note that the cervix descends on Valsalva manoeuvre almost to the level of the introitus. You take the Pap smear, which is overdue. There is a small rectocele and her perineum is somewhat deficient. The vaginal wall is atrophic. With the speculum still in situ, you ask Sandra to cough and you see a small amount of urine leak out of the urethra. You remove the speculum and when Sandra returns to the supine position, you perform a bimanual vaginal examination to check the size of the uterus and to exclude any adnexal masses. The examination is normal.

> Sandra then asks, 'So what do you think, doctor? Will that operation be suitable for me? I really don't want to undergo a larger operation. Is there anything else that can be done?'

You explain to Sandra that from your examination you believe she is experiencing mostly stress incontinence related to the presence of the prolapse. You further explain that conservative forms of therapy are worth trying. They will not 'cure' the underlying causes, but they may modify the symptoms enough that her lifestyle may improve.

Sandra asks about ring pessaries, saying that she had an aunt who used one

You explain that this is a treatment usually only reserved for elderly or infirm women where the risks of surgery are too high. The pessary, inserted by a doctor and checked every 4–6 months, when it may be changed, lies transversely in the vagina, resting behind the pubic symphysis and in the posterior fornix, thereby supporting the uterovaginal prolapse. It is not a suitable option for Sandra as she is relatively young, in good health and sexually active. You arrange a referral to a continence adviser at your hospital, as well as an MSU to exclude infection—this is reported as negative.

Conservative approach to prolapse and incontinence

- Topical oestrogen therapy will treat atrophy of the vaginal and urethral epithelium in postmenopausal women, and may result in some improvement of symptoms.
- Pelvic floor exercises explained by a trained health professional, such as a continence adviser or a physiotherapist, can result in significant improvement in prolapse and stress incontinence symptoms. Even if surgery is performed, pelvic floor exercises should be practised regularly to maintain pelvic floor muscle strength and tone.
- Bladder retraining (bladder drill) can improve symptoms of urinary urgency and urge incontinence—remember that these are not treated surgically.

Two months later you see Sandra again. *How are you getting on?* you ask her

'Doctor, I feel as if I have improved but the prolapse is still there, and I still have to wear a pad for the incontinence,' Sandra tells you. 'I think I would like to consider surgery after all.'

Does Sandra need further investigation before surgery is offered?

Yes. She should have urodynamic studies performed. Urodynamic studies are performed to confirm the diagnosis, and are mandatory before continence surgery is performed. If urine loss can be proven with coughing, in the absence of detrusor activity, this confirms the diagnosis of 'urodynamic stress incontinence'. Detrusor overactivity is confirmed by the rise of detrusor pressure at abnormally low bladder volumes. The tests are measured, recorded and adjusted by computers.

Sandra has urodynamics performed and stress incontinence is confirmed. A vaginal hysterectomy and pelvic floor repair is initially recommended by your consultant, to be followed by a suburethral tape insertion 3 months later as it is her normal practice not to perform these procedures simultaneously. Sandra agrees to this recommendation.

Clinical comment

Treatment for prolapse and incontinence

- Detrusor overactivity is treated with anticholinergic medications, such as oxybutinin and tolterodine. Side effects such as a dry mouth or blurred vision are common. It is important to advise patients that 'dry knickers may mean a dry mouth'!
- Urodynamic stress incontinence has been treated surgically with a multitude of operations. The best cure rate that can be obtained is 90%—it is most important that the patient understands this. Until recently, the 'gold standard' for this condition was a Burch colposuspension. Recently, however, suburethral tape procedures have replaced this operation, have a similar efficacy and are much simpler to perform.
- Surgery for prolapse is also varied and currently a very contentious issue. Historically, the approach has centred around various types of vaginal surgery. However, because of high recurrence rates other forms of surgery are being tried and assessed. These include abdominal approaches, laparoscopic approaches and the use of mesh as for surgical hernia repairs. Most experts agree that each case should be treated on its own merits, and may involve different approaches depending upon the individual problem. This also means that different gynaecologists may have different approaches

to the same problem, which can be confusing for the patient and the referring doctor!

Six months later you see Sandra again in the outpatients department. It is now 6 weeks since the second procedure; all has gone well with her surgery.

'I'm very happy, doctor. My prolapse is gone, and I'm much more comfortable. I'm still using the cream you gave me. I don't need to wear pads anymore, which is fantastic. I feel like I've got my life back!'

You tell Sandra you are very happy things have improved for her, and refer her back to her general practitioner, reminding her that although she no longer requires Pap smears she still needs regular mammograms.

Clinical pearls

- All women should be encouraged to perform pelvic floor exercises regularly. Women should be assessed at postnatal visits for pelvic floor strength and referred to a physiotherapist or continence adviser if instruction in how to perform pelvic floor exercises is required.
- Women who have undergone total hysterectomy (i.e. with removal of the cervix) and who have never had previous cervical abnormalities no longer require Pap smears. However, if there have been prior abnormalities with or without treatment, regular smears of the vaginal vault are recommended.

References and further reading

Dean NM, Ellis G, Wilson PD, Herbison GP. Laparoscopic colposuspension for urinary incontinence in women. Cochrane Database Syst Rev 2006; 3:CD002239.

Hart SR, Moore RD, Miklos JR, Mattox TF, Kohli N. Incidence of concomitant surgery for pelvic organ prolapse in patients surgically treated for stress urinary incontinence. J Reprod Med 2006; 51(7):521–4.

Ho MH, Lin LL, Haessler AL, Bhatia NN. Tension-free transobturator tape procedure for stress urinary incontinence. Curr Opin Obstet Gynecol 2006; 18(5):567–74.

Kobashi KC, Kobashi LI. Female stress urinary incontinence: review of the current literature. Minerva Ginecol 2006; 58(4):265–82.

Royal College of Obstetricians and Gynaecologists. Clinical Green-top Guidelines: Urodynamic Stress Incontinence—Surgical Treatment. Available online at www.rcog.org.uk.

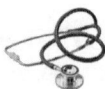

Multiple choice questions and answers

Advice for answering multiple choice questions

The following is advice for answering multiple choice questions (MCQs) in undergraduate and postgraduate examinations at the level of the Diplomas of the Royal Colleges of Obstetrics and Gynaecology.

All MCQs have a stem and, usually, five possible answers. In the following set of 30 MCQs, only *one* answer is correct. Other methods of multiple choice questioning include having only one answer which is incorrect, or a mixture of correct and incorrect answers which need to be marked true or false respectively.

However, in answering MCQs the same techniques should always be applied. Firstly, read the stem and be absolutely certain you understand the question. If you are uncertain, re-read the stem as you look down each possible answer and relate the answer to the question. Carefully consider negative statements—and particularly those where double negatives are used, which should occur only rarely. Remember, the aim of the examination is to assess whether you have a good general knowledge of the principles of the main topics and a specific understanding of important points, especially those concerned with patient safety. Examiners generally tend to set straightforward questions with straightforward answers—they are not deliberately trying to trick you. As you consider your answers, give some thought generally to the topic the examiner is questioning you on.

Work through the questions you are sure about and come back to the others later. If there is negative marking, consider how many points you may stand to lose if you guess or half-guess answers. This may be the difference between passing and failing.

Good luck!

Questions

1. A 24-year-old primigravid woman at 32 weeks' gestation presents to a small rural hospital 80 km from the base hospital with 2–3 regular contractions every 10 minutes. The CTG is normal. Speculum examination shows a slightly open, fully effaced cervix. Which of the following statements is correct?

   A Steroids should not be given because the pregnancy has already reached 32 weeks.

   B There is no point in giving tocolytics because labour is already established.

   C She should be given nifedipine and transferred by road ambulance to the base hospital.

   D She should be observed over 4 hours to determine if labour is becoming established.

   E She should have the membranes ruptured to ascertain whether meconium liquor is present.

2. A 20-year-old woman presents with severe bilateral lower abdominal pain of 12 hours duration and a temperature of 39.9°C. What is the most likely diagnosis?

   A Appendicitis

   B Urinary tract infection

   C Pelvic inflammatory disease

   D Diverticulitis

   E Pelvic thrombosis

3. Which of the following is true of the NHMRC guidelines for cervical screening in Australia?

   A All women should undergo annual Pap smears between the ages of 20 and 65.

   B Women with a report of a low-grade squamous intraepithelial lesion (LSIL) should be referred immediately for colposcopy.

   C Women with a positive Pap smear report, whether LSIL or HSIL, should have testing for high-risk HPV types.

   D A Pap smear should be performed on every woman presenting with chlamydial infection regardless of when the last Pap smear was performed.

   E Women with a report of possible HSIL should be referred immediately for colposcopy.

4. A 31-year-old Aboriginal Australian woman presents at about 7 months pregnant to a rural health centre, having had no antenatal care to date. She has had five previous full-term pregnancies. She has had an episode of moderate vaginal bleeding which was not accompanied by any pain. Your immediate management should be:

    A transfer by air to the nearest hospital
    B monitoring of vital signs and presence of fetal heart
    C speculum examination to determine the cause of the bleeding
    D bimanual vaginal examination to determine the cause of bleeding
    E coagulation screen

5. In a woman presenting with vulval pruritus in general practice:

    A inspection of the vulva and referral of any woman with signs of lichen sclerosus or ulceration should be the first line of treatment
    B empirical treatment with steroids and/or topical oestrogen should be the first line of treatment
    C the general practitioner should biopsy any suspicious looking lesion
    D lichen sclerosus can be diagnosed on inspection only
    E vulval intraepithelial neoplasia (low-grade or high-grade lesions) can be diagnosed on inspection only

6. A painless lower abdominal swelling in a girl of 16 with a negative β-HCG test is most likely to be:

    A pelvic kidney
    B hydrosalpinx
    C endometrioma
    D benign ovarian cyst
    E faecal impaction

7. Which of the following statements is true in regard to endometriosis?

    A The most common sites are the ovary and the pouch of Douglas.
    B Symptoms are directly related to the size of the lesions.
    C A diagnosis can be made on the basis of symptoms only.
    D In older women the best treatment is to wait for the onset of the menopause.
    E Oestrogen-only hormone therapy should be given immediately following hysterectomy and bilateral oophorectomy for pelvic endometriosis to reduce the risk of menopausal symptoms.

8. A LLETZ procedure (large loop excision of the transformation zone):

   A is always performed under general anaesthesia

   B should be followed up with a further Pap smear after 1 year

   C is successful at removing the lesion in about 60% of cases

   D is commonly followed by vaginal bleeding or discharge for 7–10 days

   E can frequently interfere with cervical function and the woman's subsequent chances of pregnancy

9. Genuine stress incontinence of urine:

   A does not occur in conjunction with urge incontinence

   B is not helped by pelvic floor exercises

   C is not generally helped by lifestyle measures

   D must have urodynamic studies undertaken before surgical treatment is offered

   E is best treated with anticholinergic drugs

10. Dysfunctional uterine bleeding:

   A can be diagnosed by history alone of regular heavy periods

   B often responds well to the use of the levonorgestrel-releasing IUCD

   C can be diagnosed by pipelle sampling (endometrial biopsy) alone

   D is always associated with anovulatory bleeding

   E should never be treated with the COCP

11. In conducting management of low-risk spontaneous labour, which of the following is correct?

   A Continuous fetal monitoring by CTG reduces the incidence of perinatal mortality and morbidity.

   B An intravenous line should be established early in labour in case of sudden emergency.

   C An oxytocic should be offered routinely at the end of the second stage to reduce the incidence of postpartum haemorrhage.

   D Oxytocics routinely are not indicated and the placenta should always be left to deliver spontaneously (a physiological third stage).

   E Continuous fetal monitoring reduces the incidence of caesarean section.

12. In ovarian cancer:

A overall survival rate is good, with about 75% having 5-year survival

B pain is a common early presenting symptom

C postcoital bleeding is an early symptom

D laparotomy, debulking and chemotherapy is the most common first-line treatment

E there is no familial tendency

13. A 27-year-old woman presents 6 weeks following her LMP with left iliac fossa pain and slight postcoital bleeding. A urinary β-HCG test is positive. Which of the following is correct?

A No vaginal examination should be performed until ultrasound scan has established that the placenta is not low-lying.

B Ultrasound is not useful at distinguishing intra- from extrauterine pregnancy at this gestation.

C Serial β-HCGs at weekly intervals are the most accurate way of making a diagnosis.

D Speculum examination should be carried out to check the cervical appearance and dilatation.

E Methotrexate should be given if a fetal heart is not seen on ultrasound.

14. A 35-year-old woman presents at 8 weeks in her third pregnancy. Her last pregnancy was complicated by diet-controlled gestational diabetes mellitus (GDM). Which of the following is true?

A Fetal morphology ultrasound scan and glucose tolerance testing should both be performed at 18 weeks' gestation.

B She should be commenced on oral hypoglycaemics.

C She is not at an increased risk of GDM in this pregnancy.

D Glucose tolerance testing should be performed at 24–28 weeks of pregnancy.

E There is no increased risk of fetal abnormality above that of the general population.

15. A 28-year-old woman presents with 7 weeks amenorrhoea, severe abdominal pain, worse in the lower abdomen, and slight vaginal bleeding. Her blood pressure is 90/55 mmHg, pulse rate is 110 bpm, she is afebrile, and a urinary β-HCG test is positive. Which statement is correct?

A The most likely diagnosis is ruptured appendix.

B The most likely diagnosis is ruptured spleen.

C Urgent laparoscopy and possible laparotomy for possible ruptured ectopic pregnancy is indicated.

D Ultrasound scan of the abdomen should be performed before making a decision about treatment.

E The woman should be consented for possible hysterectomy.

16. A 30-year-old nulliparous woman presents requesting laparoscopic sterilisation. Her weight is 100 kg and she has had a previous open cholecystectomy. Her current contraceptive method is the COCP. Your counselling should include which of the following statements?

    A There is no contraindication to the procedure being performed laparoscopically as only the lower abdomen is involved.

    B Her partner should give his consent to the procedure.

    C She should be quite certain she will not wish to have children in the future.

    D There will be no change in her menstrual cycles after the procedure.

    E The procedure is easily reversible.

17. An 18-year-old nulliparous woman presents asking for effective contraception. She has been prescribed the COCP but has trouble remembering to take it. Which of the following statements is likely to be most applicable to her situation?

    A Condoms are highly effective and also will protect against STIs.

    B The etonogestrel rod is highly effective and once in place requires no patient action for 3 years.

    C Intramuscular medroxyprogesterone acetate is highly effective and is given every 3 months but may cause unpredictable heavy bleeding.

    D A copper-bearing IUCD can be inserted and remain in place for 5 years but may be associated with heavy periods.

    E Taking an active pill every day with no break for withdrawal bleeds may be easier to manage.

18. Spontaneous preterm labour may be due to:

    A previous caesarean section

    B previous multiple pregnancy

    C previous large baby

    D pyelonephritis

    E monilial (*Candida*) infection

19. A 36-year-old woman underwent emergency caesarean section for fetal distress in her first pregnancy. She is now 20 weeks advanced in the second pregnancy and seeks advice about delivery on this occasion. Which of the following statements is true?

A A first caesarean section should always be followed by a repeat caesarean in the next pregnancy.

B A first caesarean section should always be followed by an attempt at vaginal birth.

C Risks of haemorrhage and organ damage with caesarean section on this occasion are exactly the same as on the first occasion.

D The risks of both repeat caesarean section and attempted vaginal birth should be outlined to her.

E She should have tubal ligation performed with a second caesarean section because the risks from a third caesarean are very high.

20. Severe hyperemesis gravidarum:

A always requires admission to hospital

B always requires termination of the pregnancy

C occurs in 1 in 100 pregnancies

D is always psychosomatic in origin

E is not associated with multiple pregnancy

21. A 20-year-old woman presents at 36 weeks of pregnancy with recurrent herpes genitalis (HSV-2) infection on the perineum. Which of the following statements is true?

A Aciclovir or valaciclovir administration from 36 weeks to delivery will reduce the chances of a further outbreak at the time of delivery.

B Immediate caesarean section is indicated.

C Elective caesarean section at 38 weeks gestation is indicated.

D HSV-2 commonly crosses the placenta close to term and may cause intrauterine encephalitis.

E HSV-2 poses no risk at all to the baby in a recurrent episode.

22. Placental abruption:

A always presents with vaginal bleeding

B is more common in primigravidae than in multiparae

C is a potential complication of attempted external cephalic version for breech presentation

D is not more common in twin pregnancy

E is never an indication for caesarean section

23. A 30-year-old woman with type 1 diabetes is in the 37th week of her first pregnancy. Blood sugar levels are well controlled. Which of the following statements is true?

A Caesarean section should be performed at 38 weeks.

B Induction of labour should be planned for a mutually acceptable time between 38 and 40 weeks.

C She can be allowed to continue past 40 weeks and until 42 weeks awaiting spontaneous labour.

D At this gestation the infant is not at risk of respiratory distress syndrome.

E At this gestation the infant is not at risk of hypoglycaemia.

24. A 33-year-old woman presents seeking advice—she has had three consecutive first trimester miscarriages. Which of the following statements is true?

A Recurrent miscarriage occurs in about 15–20% of women in the reproductive age group.

B Bed rest may help prevent recurrent miscarriage.

C The chances of successful full-term pregnancy after one miscarriage is less than 50%.

D Recurrent miscarriage may be prevented by taking 150 mg aspirin daily.

E The cause of most cases of recurrent miscarriage is usually not identifiable.

25. The levonorgestrel-releasing IUCD:

A is contraindicated for a breastfeeding woman

B must be removed or changed after 2 years

C is not suitable for a postmenopausal woman taking oral oestrogen hormone therapy

D can be used as a method of emergency contraception up to a week following unprotected intercourse

E is not contraindicated after one previous caesarean section

26. Rhesus negative women who become pregnant:

A do not need to be given anti-D prophylaxis after early miscarriage (before 8 weeks)

B do not need to be given anti-D prophylaxis following early surgical abortion (before 8 weeks)

C should be tested for antibodies on at least two occasions during a continuing pregnancy

D should be given anti-D prophylaxis after delivery even if the baby is Rhesus positive

E should not be offered external cephalic version if the baby presents as a breech

27. A 30-year-old woman in her fourth pregnancy has a history of severe shoulder dystocia in the last delivery, causing a third-degree tear. She seeks advice about the current pregnancy and mode of delivery. Which of the following statements is true?

A She should plan a vaginal birth but elective episiotomy should be performed.

B Another third-degree tear properly repaired does not increase her subsequent risk of pelvic floor dysfunction.

C Glucose tolerance testing may be performed but will not influence the mode of delivery.

D Elective caesarean section should be discussed with her.

E Vaginal birth should be attempted with the possibility of emergency caesarean section if progress is slow.

28. Breech presentation:

A occurs in about 10% of full-term pregnancies

B is not associated with fetal abnormality

C is associated with a higher perinatal mortality and morbidity than cephalic presentation

D is not more common in preterm infants

E is not more common in twins

29. A 38-year-old woman gravida 4, three previous full-term vaginal deliveries, presents at 36 weeks of pregnancy with headache, blurring of vision and ankle swelling. She has a history of hypertension prior to the pregnancy. Ward testing of urine reveals +3 of protein. Your management is likely to include:

A   weekly ultrasound scans to assess fetal growth over the next
     4 weeks
B   prescribing increased doses of her oral hypertensive therapy
C   antibiotics for probable urinary tract infection
D   immediate caesarean section
E   admission to hospital and early induction of labour

30. You are arranging admission and operation for a 30-year-old woman
having a planned repeat caesarean section. She has had two previous
caesarean sections. Which of the following statements is true?

A   It is not necessary to describe the risks of the surgery to her
     because she has had the operation twice before and knows all
     about it.
B   You advise her that it is likely general anaesthesia will be used.
C   A third caesarean section is commonly associated with excessive
     blood loss so blood will be cross-matched and you advise her that
     transfusion is very likely.
D   You advise her that the risk of damage to bowel and/or bladder is
     no greater than with her previous caesarean sections.
E   It is appropriate to discuss with her the possibility of tubal ligation
     being performed in conjunction with the caesarean.

Answers

1. C	**11.** C	**21.** A
2. C	**12.** D	**22.** C
3. E	**13.** D	**23.** B
4. B	**14.** A	**24.** C
5. A	**15.** C	**25.** E
6. D	**16.** C	**26.** C
7. A	**17.** B	**27.** D
8. D	**18.** D	**28.** C
9. D	**19.** D	**29.** E
10. B	**20.** A	**30.** E

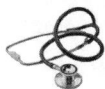

Index